THE

BOOZE CHEESE

AND

CHOCOLATE

DIET

ISBN: 978-0-6450566-6-2 (paperback)
ISBN: 978-0-6450566-7-9 (ebook)

Published by Bouley Bay Books, Sydney & Jersey
Tel: (+61) 403 039 164
Email: MLM444@gmail.com
Typeset & printed in Australia by Image DTO
Tel: (+61) 423 360 883 imagedto@gmail.com
Cover Design and illustrations by Trish Le Moignan

First published 2022
www.bouleybaybooks.com

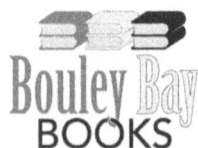

Bouley Bay
BOOKS

The Booze, Cheese and Chocolate Diet

How to Lose Weight
without Misery
and
How to Lower Cholesterol Levels
without Statins

by Mick le Moignan
with additional advice by
Dr Naras Lapsys, Consultant Dietitian
and
Mr William Shakespeare, Playwright

Illustrated by Trish Le Moignan

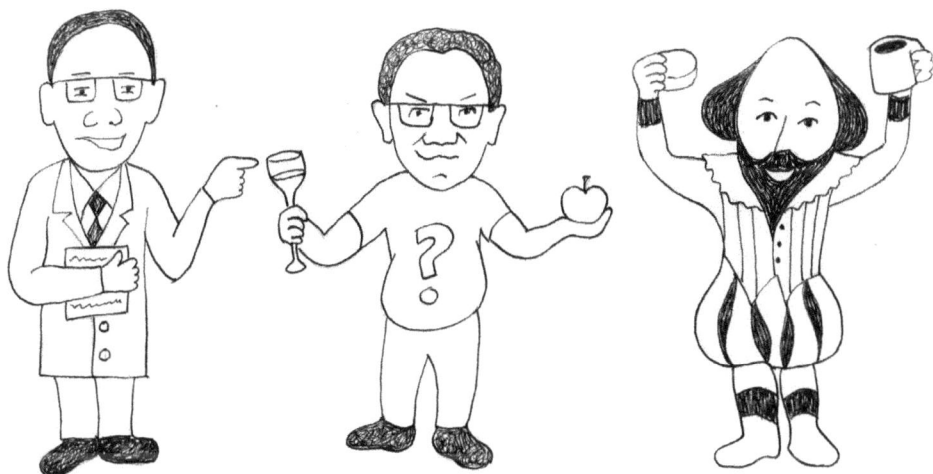

When you look
in your mirror
who do you see?

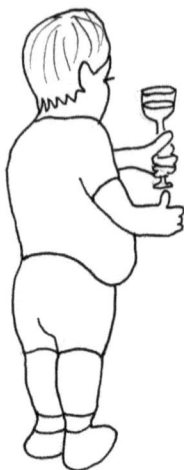

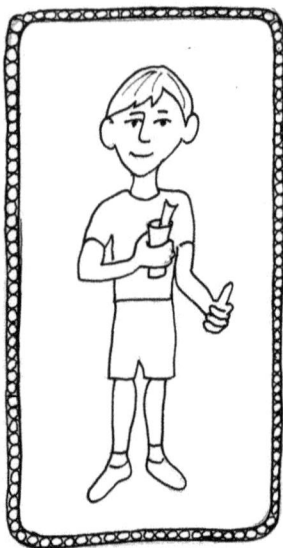

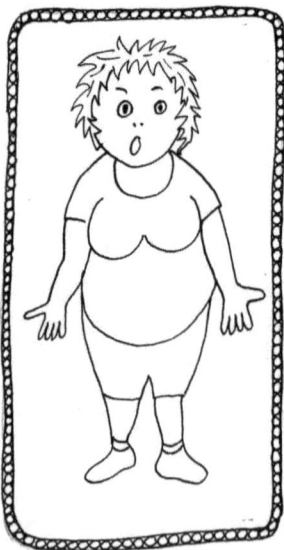

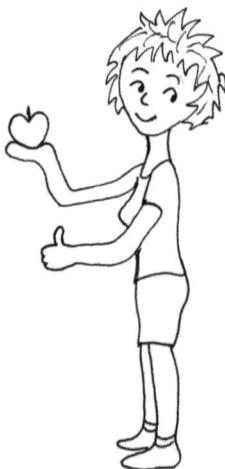

Contents

Foreword

Congratulations! Whether you bought, begged, borrowed or stole this book – or, better still, if you received it as a gift from a kind and caring friend or relation – you are clearly a person who appreciates the finer pleasures of life. You are not afraid to luxuriate in the delights of the three demons of all diets, alcohol, cheese and chocolate. You may be modest in your indulgence – or reckless to a fault. You may not yet be a card-carrying, fully fledged hedonist, but you have probably passed some of the preliminary tests and you are on the road to – to what?

I hate to suggest this, but you may be on the way to being a fat drunk with spots and smelly breath, for that is where over-indulgence leads. Booze, cheese and chocolate are miracles of human ingenuity. People say 'You can't have too much of a good thing' but it's not true. You can. On the other hand, cutting out these good things altogether would be a pointless sacrifice: it would amount to chucking out the chocolate untasted, the cheese uncut and the wine still in its bottle.

'Moderation in all things' is an admirable ideal – but terribly dull. 'Moderation in all things, including moderation' is the way to go, because limiting moderation allows for those glorious break-outs, the times when you consume too much of something and simply don't care – until the next morning, when you wake up feeling as if the Rusty Nail cocktails that were so delicious last night were actually hammered into your head.

Or maybe you catch sight of a podgy person in the bathroom mirror and dismiss the thought that it might be you – until you notice that the bathroom scales are registering an extra kilo or three – again.

How to indulge in pleasure with impunity is the puzzle this book sets out to solve. Naturally, it involves some checks and balances, some restraint and some monitoring of one's intake – but not so much as to kill the joy. On the contrary, the aim is to show you how to take even more delight in the ecstatic experiences offered by chocolate, cheese, wine, beer and mood-enhancing spirits, while helping you to avoid unappealing pitfalls, such as diabetes, obesity, cirrhosis of the liver and premature death.

If you want to lose weight and/or lower your cholesterol levels, there is no need to suffer the pain and inconvenience of crucifying yourself along the way: here is a simple roadmap that will guide you on the path to a slimmer, fitter, younger-looking, younger-feeling and more desirable YOU!

'This above all: to thine own self be true,
And it must follow, as the night the day,
Thou canst not then be false to any man.'

Polonius' advice to his son, Laertes, in *Hamlet*,
Act 1, Scene 3,
by William Shakespeare.

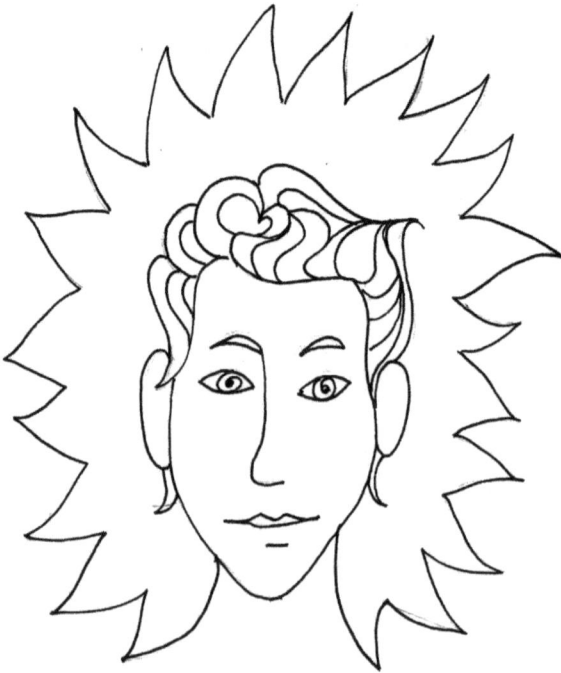

Chapter 1

What do you want to achieve?

Nobody sets out on a journey without some idea of where they want to go – and it's exactly the same with dieting. You will only succeed if you first work out what your ultimate goal is and then set a time-frame for your journey to success.

If you're a very brave, gregarious, outgoing sort of person, you can try telling all your partners, lovers, children, colleagues, friends and neighbours that you've decided to lose weight. The upside of that approach is that you will have engaged your pride and nailed your colours to the mast: they will watch you closely over the next few days and weeks, to see how you go. That may help to motivate you.

The downside is that, if you fail to make the rapid progress you intend, they will probably mock you. You will feel like an alpine skier who has missed a slalom gate; you'll try too hard to recover your balance and end up face-down and covered with shame in a metaphorical snowdrift. If you are really brave and outgoing (see above), you'll just dust yourself off and start again – and good luck to you, because you'll need it.

For the rest of us, a less public, more circumspect approach is safer. Professional fundraisers, embarking on a capital appeal to raise, say, $100 million, make sure they have secured at least half of their target funds before they announce the start of the 'public phase' of the campaign. That way, they don't risk losing face or crashing into a metaphorical snowdrift. However, it is vital to set and declare a goal of some sort. The prudent course is to put it in writing, so that your Other Self cannot fudge the figures later or persuade you to forget what your True Self intended.

Sadly, where dieting is concerned, we all have an incredible capacity for self-deception. Think of it as a battle between your different selves, two aspects of your personality. Your brain wants you to be slim, svelte, fit and attractive. Your belly wants to be filled with food and drink. The brain is clever but the belly is crafty: it has many devious ways of persuading you to give it what it wants. Your belly pretends to be starving, in desperate need of sustenance, just to keep going. It uses your senses to remind you how delicious things taste, how much fun you have when you give it what it wants. The poor brain, with only cold logic and common sense, is often powerless against this sensual onslaught, at least until the next morning, when the damage done is all too apparent.

Your Two Selves

Let's be brutally honest and call these two sides your True Self and your Greedy Self. Your Greedy Self is the source of much pleasure: you're not going to deny it forever, but you will enjoy those pleasures even more if you allow your True Self to take charge and make some key choices for you. You really can have the best of both selves, but at times, this will require strong willpower and determination. Your brain knows best. You can do this – and the more firmly and frequently you assert your will, the easier it will become. The reward will be a massive change in your life – from transient pleasures to long-lasting happiness.

If you're serious about losing weight – and if you're not, why are you still reading this? – it's a huge help to record your progress. Weigh yourself EVERY DAY and write it down. Either open a new file or folder on your computer, marking it 'For Your Eyes Only' or buy a small notebook, if you prefer a hard copy. Or use the progress charts thoughtfully provided for that very purpose at the end of this book. Start by writing down your target weight – in an ideal world. Then choose your target date – some future day by which you hope to achieve your goal. If you have tried in the past to lose weight, think back and write a few notes about those experiences. Treat them like a private diary: they are for your benefit, no-one else's. So tell yourself the truth. Pull no punches.

What were you trying to achieve? Did you succeed? Did you lose some weight and put it on again afterwards? Why do you think that happened? What are some of the setbacks you will try to avoid, this time? And – perhaps above all – why are you doing this to yourself? Do you really want to improve your health and fitness, or is it just a passing fantasy?

The notebook is only for your guidance, so you may as well be as honest as you can. We all tend to repeat our mistakes, but remembering them may help you to avoid them, down the track. Our Greedy Self is brilliant at pulling the wool over our eyes. Look that fat person in the mirror firmly in the eye and tell them who's boss. It's for their own good. A slimmer person will thank you later for your strength of character.

If you plan to reduce your weight by a substantial amount, break the task into manageable chunks or phases. The workers who built the Great Wall of China were asked to construct relatively small sections at a time: when they had completed them, they were rewarded and sent home for a well-earned rest. Of course, there was a master plan, but it would have been too daunting and dispiriting for them to keep it in mind all the time.

One Question

You are not building a Wall, but there will be many times when it will help you to concentrate on the immediate task, rather than risk overwhelming yourself with the difficulties involved in reaching your goal. Typically, that immediate task will be one simple decision:

'Am I going to eat/drink this – or not?'

You make this decision over and over again, every day of your life. It's not to be taken lightly and certainly not too quickly. Give it very careful thought. Don't rely on your instincts: use your brain and try to be as present, aware and mindful as possible. Make sure your decisions are not guided by the aptly named 'gut instincts'.

For much of the time, the answer to that perennial question will need to be a very firm and determined 'NO'. However, one of the underlying principles of the Booze, Cheese and Chocolate Diet is that even small successes should be rewarded – without, of course, undermining your original achievement.

One advantage of having more manageable targets is that you will provide yourself with opportunities – indeed, cast-iron excuses – to celebrate. Yes, this is where the booze, cheese and chocolate come in. Perhaps we should agree at this stage to say this is where the booze, cheese OR chocolate comes in. Indulging in all three at a sitting should be a rare treat, reserved for super-indulgent occasions. And yes, I know how well red wine goes with cheese, we can negotiate on that.

'O, that this too, too solid flesh would melt,
Thaw and resolve itself into a dew!'
from Hamlet's soliloquy in *Hamlet*, Act 1, Scene 2,
by William Shakespeare.

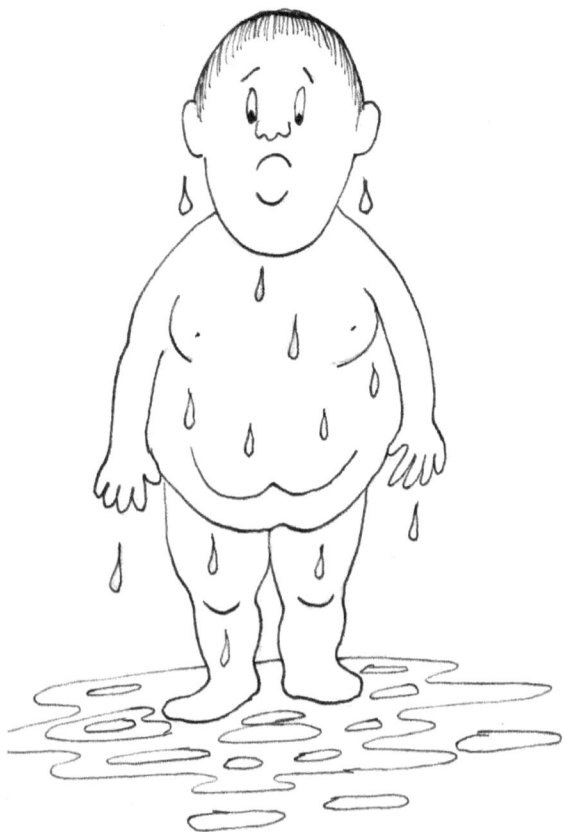

2

How much do you care?

Forgive the personal questions, but they could save us – well, you – a considerable amount of time, effort and heartache. 'No pain, no gain' is all very well, but pain without reward is pointless. Don't embark on a diet unless you are determined to see it through to the end. You will need to know yourself well, both limitations and capabilities.

Take a look at your body, naked in the bathroom mirror. What do you see? A fine figure of a man – or woman? Perhaps you observe some evidence of over-indulgence or a falling-off in physical fitness: surely, such minor imperfections could easily be concealed by canny choices of clothing – dresses that are floaty, rather than figure-hugging, informal shirts that hang outside the trousers, rather than being tucked in tightly at the bulging waistline.

Prudent dressing can cover a multitude of imperfections. It's not too difficult to conceal a moderate amount of obesity. But who are you fooling? At the end of the day, there you are, back in front of the bathroom mirror, still carrying those superfluous kilos. If you're only slightly overweight, you may decide the small deception is harmless. You're not really pretending – just trying to look your best. Or is the problem more serious than that? Are you more than generously proportioned? Actually obese, a tub of lard, filled to overflowing?

What are you prepared to do about it? To what lengths will you go, to effect the changes you require? How will you handle the excuses and counter-arguments that may sap your resolve? Perhaps this is how 'Nature' intended you to be. A little excess baggage may be embedded in your genetic code. Who are you, to go against your own DNA? You might be 'big-framed'. Have you 'always had a little puppy-fat'? Did you never quite shake off the effects of growing and nurturing your babies? Weight loss may be harder for you than for others.

Your True Self knows this is all rubbish. Prompted by the slightest hint of deprivation, your devious Greedy Self will conjure up any number of persuasive arguments to keep your snout glued to the trough. Your True Self will need to stay alert and vigilant, ready to tell your Greedy Self to shut its mouth and stop eating. Otherwise, however firmly you have made up your mind, you will find yourself standing at your fridge or larder, shovelling in food before your conscious mind has even noticed what's happening.

Never Give In

Some time after the end of the Second World War, Winston Churchill gave a memorable after-dinner speech at an Oxford college. The diners were eager to hear what the great man had to say. He stood up, glowered around and stated firmly: 'Never give in!' He left a long pause, during which he surveyed his audience and took a puff on his cigar. Then he spoke more quietly, as if imparting a valuable piece of advice: 'Never give in!' Another pause followed, even longer than the first, with another puff on his cigar, after which he pronounced with finality, as if it were the conclusion to a long and complex argument: 'Never – give in!' And he sat down to a stunned silence, quickly followed by tumultuous applause. The diners never forgot a single word of his speech.

Fortunately, you are not called upon to do battle with Nazi hordes on the beaches of Britain – but you could probably do with some of Churchill's bulldog-like determination. And you would do well to heed his advice. There will be setbacks, moments when you succumb to temptation. You will lose the occasional battle: just make sure you don't lose the war.

Later chapters will include some practical strategies for dealing with temptations, but it is worth realising from the outset that you will need to be vigilant. Your Greedy Self will seize on any moment of weakness or inattention. Learn to resist it. After a while, you'll find it can be deeply satisfying to take back control of this area of your life. You know you're right: it's for your own good. Stay on guard and be firm about it.

The personal questions above and the recommendation to take a good look at yourself naked in the bathroom mirror are not intended to disgust you or make you loathe the sight of yourself. Their purpose is simply to invite you to make an honest assessment. If you are content with your body, even if it has a little more flesh on the bones than you would like, why go to the trouble of trying to changing it? It's your decision, either way, but it should be an informed one, based on the facts.

If it's not important to you to lose weight, why bother? The energy you will expend could be used on many other activities that will bring you pleasure or satisfaction without any hardship. Don't underestimate the degree of difficulty in the change you are contemplating – but if you really do want to reduce your weight and/or lower your cholesterol levels, don't shirk the challenge, or put it off to another day. Help is at hand – in your own hands, right now, in fact – and the rewards for succeeding may include you living a longer, happier, healthier life.

Hunger can be your friend

For most people, it is much easier to add fat than to remove it. The body is reluctant to give up the stores it has set aside for a rainy day. Rather than melting down fat, it will urge you to eat – and our bodies, in the form of our Greedy Selves, can be terribly persuasive.

In steeling yourself to refuse these internal entreaties, remember that unacceptable image in the bathroom mirror. Take a photograph of it, if you like, to use as inspiration. Just be careful not to post it on social media. This is your battle and your business, no-one else's. That portly person really is you: soon, if you persevere, it may be the old you. Then you can post it on social media, if that's your bag. 'Here I am, before and after my miraculous transformation!'

If you have really decided to change your physique, stick to your guns. You may feel the occasional pang of hunger, but don't give in to it at once. Examine the sensation. Study it carefully. How bad is it, really? How long does it go on, if you ignore it?

Try drinking a cup of tea or coffee: they have few calories, if you add just a little milk, and no sugar, and will usually wash away any slight feelings of hunger. Don't be afraid of hunger pangs, in any case – welcome them! For they are a sign that your solid, sullied flesh is at last beginning to melt and thaw. Spring is on the way.

'Let me have men about me that are fat;
Sleek-headed men and such as sleep o' nights:
Yond Cassius has a lean and hungry look;
He thinks too much: such men are dangerous.'

Julius Caesar, speaking about one of his assassins.
He was right, but he didn't act in time to save his life.

in *Julius Caesar*, Act 1, Scene 3, by William Shakespeare

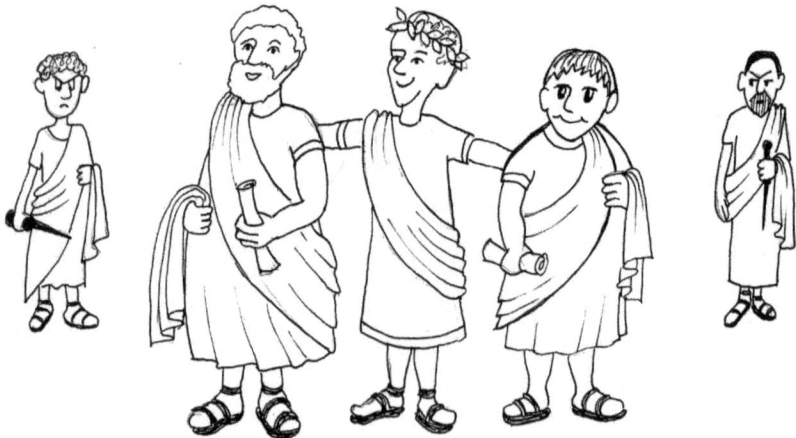

3

How hard is this going to be?

Successful dieting is not rocket science. 'Eat less, move more' just about sums it up. What goes in must come out, unless it is used as energy or stored as fat. Weight loss happens when the fat stores are not replenished as fast as they are being used.

All foods, including alcohol, contain calories, which are 'burned' by the body as it goes about its daily business. More energetic occupations, such as running, weight-lifting and other forms of exercise burn more calories and therefore allow more to be consumed. This is a dangerous concept for anyone trying to lose weight. The temptation is to let yourself eat more, simply because you are taking more exercise than usual. Like most temptations, it should be examined carefully and then resisted. After exercise, you may feel hungrier for a few moments, but that is because some of your stores of fat have been used up and the body suggests replacing them. Do you really want to do that?

The second requirement for successful dieting, after your personal diary, is a good weighing machine. Some dieticians recommend weighing yourself only once a week. If you are determined to lose weight, I believe it is much better to weigh yourself every day, as soon as you get up, before taking any liquids or solids.

This will motivate you to stay strong and will keep you up to date with your progress. There may be some slight variations, but by and large these measurements will be accurate and you should be able to observe a slow but steady reduction in your weight. Write them down in your notebook or record them in your computer file every day for future reference and encouragement. After a few weeks, you will find that, if you think back over the previous day's calorie intake and the amount of exercise you completed, you'll be able to guess with a fair degree of accuracy what your weight will be, each morning.

One popular and effective way of dieting is the '5:2' system, devised by the writer and broadcaster, Dr Michael Mosley. Participants have a normal (but sensible) eating regime for five days of each week and go on a light fast on two days of the week. Mosley defined a fasting day as a day where men consume less than 600 calories and women less than 500. His research proved that such an interruption to the body's regular routine can be beneficial in a weight loss program, partly because it breaks into your regular pattern of habit-eating – but be careful not to make up the deficit from the two fasting days over the other five days!

Plan your week

I prefer a reverse '5:2' system, where calorie intake is controlled over the five weekdays and the rules are relaxed a little at weekends. Where self-restraint is concerned, a week is a manageable amount of time. Most people are used to working through the week and looking forward to the weekend: apply the same structure to your weight loss program. If you're a shift worker, set your week to suit your own schedule, but Monday morning is a pretty good time to make a fresh start, re-set your diet regime or just resolve to do a little better in the week ahead.

You can choose whether your weekend begins on Friday evening or goes on through Sunday evening, but it should probably include only two evenings of comparative indulgence. You can, of course, exchange a weekend day or evening for a weekday one, to set you free to enjoy a special social event, but you'll need to be strict about paying it back. It's a good idea to get the extra day of reduced intake 'in the bank' first, before loosening your belt for the celebration. If you decide to cheat, ask yourself who you're cheating.

So, decide for yourself whether your Sunday evening is going to be a case of 'Eat, drink and be merry, for tomorrow we diet' – or a chance to start focusing on tightening your belt for the week ahead. Either way can be effective: work out which suits you best.

Later chapters will include suggestions on which foods to include in your diet, but the Booze, Cheese and Chocolate Diet is not going to boss you around. We know one size doesn't fit all. You have every right to decide what you want to eat. Quality is important, but quantity control is the key. The first step is to work out what total calorie intake you can allow yourself, on a daily and weekly basis, to achieve your target weight in the time you have chosen.

If you'd like help with this, go to thebodydoctor.com.au – the website of consultant dietitian, Dr Naras Lapsys. Enter your age, gender, weight, approximate fitness level, your target weight and target date, and you will receive advice on the amount of calories per day/week you can allow yourself in order to reach your goal in the time-frame you have specified.

For more detailed help and advice on improving your overall health and lifestyle choices, Dr Lapsys offers consultations to individuals or couples, either online or in person in Sydney and Singapore, tailored to individual needs. He is 'committed to helping people obtain the knowledge, skills and motivation to make lasting changes to their health and life'.

Don't be too hard on yourself

Ease yourself into the first week. Remember that you've embarked on a marathon, not a sprint, and you don't want to collapse in a heap at the first drinks station, because you have set yourself too hard a target.

It may take a while for your stomach to adjust to a reduced intake of calories, so be gentle but firm with it. If you feel hungry, have a glass of water or a cup of tea or coffee (always without sugar and adding the minimum amount of milk to make it palatable for you) and see how you feel after twenty minutes.

If you're still hungry, eat a few nuts or seeds: the figures on your bathroom scales will tell you whether such indulgences are undermining your plan. But beware of giving in to hunger pangs too easily: a little food or a 'sugar hit' can stimulate your digestive juices and make you feel hungrier. In the long run, it may be better to learn to say 'NO' to your importunate belly.

'There was a time when all the body's members
Rebelled against the belly, thus accused it:
That only like a gulf it did remain
In the midst of the body, idle and inactive,
Still cupboarding the viand, never bearing
Like labour with the rest, where the other instruments
Did see and hear, devise, instruct, walk, feel,
And, mutually participate, did minister
Unto the appetite and affection common
Of the whole body.'
Menenius Agrippa, addressing rebellious Roman citizens
in *Coriolanus* Act 1, Scene 1, by William Shakespeare

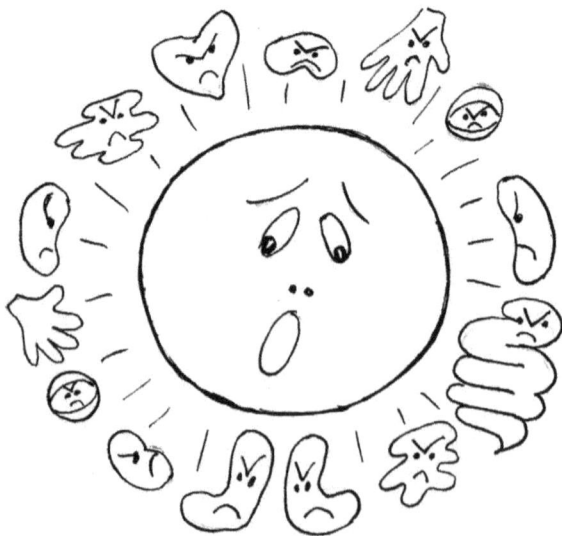

4

Are you having second thoughts or second helpings?

Going on a diet can feel revolutionary. It can provoke what may feel like an internal rebellion, if you are not used to limiting your calorie intake. There is no need to force matters: it's not a war, but a readjustment of priorities. Your True Self and your Greedy Self will need to agree on a common goal: this is their masterplan to achieve a weight loss that both can agree to be in their common interest. When the going gets tough, as it will, your two selves will need to set up an occasional summit meeting where they will engage in diplomatic negotiations and reach some sensible compromises, always bearing in mind the overall goal.

Small victories can be sweet. In the first week, a few adjustments to your regular routine may help you to achieve a pleasing initial weight loss. This can come about simply as a result of you being more conscious of what you consume. But beware. Your Greedy Self is not above the old, smoke and mirrors trick of distracting you with flattery while it force-feeds you. Our busy lives are partly to blame. We all tend to take a quick pit-stop on the run, succumbing to small temptations without really noticing what we are doing.

'Food to go' is the food that goes just where you don't want it to go. As ladies who like a cream-cake with their morning coffee learn, ruefully: 'A moment on the lips, a lifetime on the hips'.

Here's a strong recommendation: try to eat and drink mindfully. They are great pleasures. You have decided to impose some limitations on them, for the sake of your health and wellbeing. So, make sure you enjoy everything you eat and drink to the max. Don't grab snacks on the run, at the service station or standing in front of the fridge. If you are going to eat something, make it a conscious decision. Question yourself about it: do I really need this? Is this hamburger and fries going to be as delicious and desirable in five or ten minutes' time, when I have gulped it down and washed it away with a cup of sub-standard coffee or a sugary drink?

If you do decide to eat something, PUT IT ON A PLATE! Look at it. Enjoy it. Decide whether it's a friend or a foe. Ask yourself if you have too much on your plate. If so, don't be afraid to put some back, or aside. If you change your mind, you can always come back for seconds. Taste it. Savour it. Indulge your senses. Be slow to swallow, because that's the end of it. That's when the greedy belly sets your eyes and fingers on to search for more, and you may not need any more. Especially if what you have just swallowed has not yet reached your stomach.

Slow food

Fast food is generally a bad idea. Most fast food contains too many undesirable elements, like salt, sugar, saturated fats and other processed ingredients. It is rarely prepared with the love and care your meal deserves. The only argument in its favour is convenience: it saves you time to spend on other activities. Even the term 'fast food' is dangerous, because it encourages you to gulp it down without thinking too much about it. But the 'fast' refers to the preparation time. The convenience is principally for the people selling it. It's no accident that it leaves you unsatisfied, wanting more: that way, the fast food merchants can maximise their profits by selling you a second helping.

Food is more important than the fast food outlets understand. There's no rush, or there shouldn't be. If you're busy or in a hurry, just eat later. Take your time. And take it easy. No-one is going to snatch the food from your plate. You're not at boarding school, swallowing it down as quickly as you can, so you can be at the front of the line for seconds.

If you're eating less, to reduce your weight, give yourself a treat by really enjoying what you do eat. Pause between courses – or even between mouthfuls. If you're in the habit of eating fast, try really hard to slow it down. Don't be afraid to tell your belly to wait for a few minutes. Otherwise you may find yourself responding to an urgent appeal that is actually out of date, because food is already on the way to your digestive system – which will also thank you for taking your time.

Don't eat like a dog. They woof it down, barely tasting anything, and as soon as they've finished, they start looking round for more. If you tend to eat too fast, try to work out why. It's probably not hunger, but habit. And the faster you eat, the more likely you are to overeat. You can't control the size of your portion if it disappears as fast as a dog's dinner. What you call hunger pangs will subside, if you give them time. Ask yourself if you have ever been genuinely hungry, as millions of people in less fortunate nations know hunger. How often has hunger limited any of your activities? Most of the time, our fear of 'hunger' is just an excuse to stuff in more food that we don't need.

Food is love. Preparing it for someone you care about is one of the most eloquent ways of showing what you feel about them. Enjoy the elements of ritual and allow yourself to savour the moment. Food is no longer a matter of survival – but some Stone Age instincts linger on. They lure us into storing fat in our bodies in case of future shortages. For most of us, fortunately, famine is unlikely to strike, at least in the immediate future.

Remember your goal

In the hurly burly of life, it's easy to forget that you've set yourself a serious target to lose weight and improve your health and longevity. Your Greedy Self will try to kid you that you're feeling tired and need sustenance 'to keep you going'. Try to make sure your True Self vets any such requests quite carefully.

Are you really tired or just a bit bored? Tasting something sweet might relieve the tedium of a task. My father used to say 'A cup of tea is just too wet without a biscuit!' The truth is that a cup of tea or coffee is just too fattening, if you always have something to eat with it. And who wants to look like a biscuit barrel?

Losing weight will involve changing some deeply ingrained habits. You will need to be constantly vigilant, to make sure you don't slip back into old ways, without thinking. If you decide you really do deserve an indulgence, like a chocolate biscuit with your morning coffee, have one – it's your choice – but think about it, know what you're doing, make it a conscious decision, rather than succumbing to a whim, and above all, enjoy it!

This is a change of direction, not a war. Be disciplined – if you're not, your diet will go on forever – but beyond that, be gentle with yourself. What you are doing is in your best interests. The aim is to make your life longer and more enjoyable. Imagine how it would feel to climb a steep hill or a few flights of stairs carrying significantly less weight. Piling on a few extra kilos slows down even the fittest racehorses. Imagine what your self-imposed handicap is doing to you, every day. It's time to shed the load and feel lighter and brighter.

'Your most grave belly was deliberate,
Not rash like his accusers, and thus answered:
'True it is, my incorporate friends,' quoth he,
'That I receive the general food at first,
Which you do live upon; and fit it is,
Because I am the store-house and the shop
Of the whole body: but, if you do remember,
I send it through the rivers of your blood,
Even to the court, the heart, to the seat of the brain;
And, through the cranks and offices of man,
The strongest nerves and small inferior veins
From me receive that natural competency
Whereby they live.'
The belly's reply, borrowed from Aesop's Fables,
in *Coriolanus* Act 1, Scene 1, by William Shakespeare

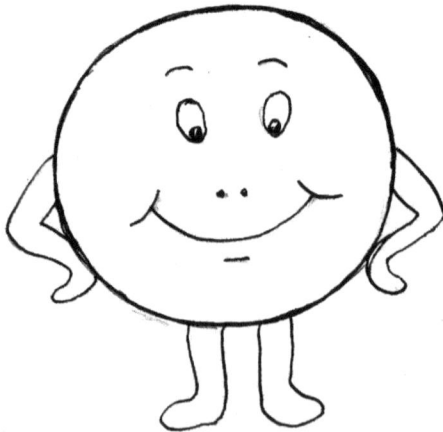

5

When can you start?

Enough exhortations and threats. As you have read this far, my guess is that you have got the point and made up your mind to do whatever it takes to succeed.

Some people think they only need to adjust their regular diet by a few degrees, in order to lose weight. They reason that, if they just cut back a little, cut down on a few fattening items and maybe take slightly smaller portions, they will reach their ideal weight without too much difficulty.

Then, they reason, it will simply be a matter of continuing their new regime, to stay at their desired weight. This is a fallacy: it doesn't take account of human nature. We love variety. If we take the fun out of food and make our meals dull and routine, we will rebel. We will break out of the dietary straitjacket and go on a binge.

We will, of course, feel guilty afterwards and try to go back to our original plan – but if it only reduces our weight slowly, we may reach the next binge long before we arrive at our ideal weight. That way, the dietary restrictions have to go on forever. No wonder that method doesn't work. This is why most people who try to lose weight give up before achieving their goals.

Instead of having one eating plan that goes on forever, it's best to have three totally different plans and vary them according to your own needs and life style.

The first plan should be a reducing diet plan, which you use to lose the weight you have decided is surplus to your requirements. It will need to be sharp enough to make a difference in a reasonable time-frame – that is, before you get bored with it and abandon it. If you're going to go to all the trouble of restricting your intake of food and drink, which will require a considerable exercise of will-power, you will want to see some significant results in the bathroom mirror.

Your reducing diet should not be a punishment, but a source of delight. Choose the foods you most like to eat. If they are loaded with calories, you will only be able to eat small quantities. Can you cope with that? Or would you prefer to choose foods that are slightly less attractive to you, but more filling and sustaining? Everyone will have their own answers – but we all need to ask ourselves the same questions.

A reducing diet plan that is perfect for YOU

We all have slightly different tastes and preferences. Few people enjoy following a rigid regime set by someone else. The Booze, Cheese and Chocolate Diet is designed, above all, to be adaptable. You're in charge. You decide what you want to eat, to balance your desire to regulate your weight and yet to enjoy your food and drink.

The purpose is to work out a daily routine that suits you and that you will be able to continue for as long as it takes, to achieve your target weight. The first requirement of your reducing diet is to make a significant reduction in your total intake of calories from all sources, but it also needs to reflect your personality and take into account your own distinctive likes and dislikes.

Start by telling your notebook a little bit about yourself.

Do you really need three square meals a day? Would three modest meals a day be enough, or could you make do with two? If so, which ones? There is a popular belief that 'breakfast is the most important meal of the day'. That may be so, because the system has longer to digest the food. By the same token, for someone seeking to lose weight, breakfast may be the best meal to cut down on or do without altogether. The hearty breakfaster may be able to skip lunch or dinner – even both. For myself, if I have a good breakfast, my belly thinks the good times are back. I'm ready for lunch and ravenous for dinner. It all depends on the chemistry and preferences of each individual, and it's vitally important to work out what yours are and act accordingly.

For me, it's relatively easy to postpone eating till lunchtime. I'm ready for something then, but if I'm busy or otherwise distracted, I can keep going till dinnertime, maybe with a low-calorie smoothie, a piece of fruit or a handful of nuts. I wasn't always that way – and bacon and eggs is still my idea of heaven on a plate – but practice helps and that works for me. Your reducing diet will only achieve your goal if you work out a regime that suits YOU.

That applies to the way you structure your week, as well. Treat each week as a separate unit. Whatever you ate or drank last week, it's too late to fix it now, so don't beat yourself up about it. Every Monday morning is a fresh start: you have a new budget of calories to spend over the next seven days, so see if you can eat and drink within your allowance, this week, or maybe even put some aside for a rainy day.

Don't be too hard on yourself

The average calorie intake varies according to your gender and how active you are, but is around 2,500 a day for men and 2,000 for women. For a reducing diet, your daily budget is likely to be about 1,500 calories for men or 1,200 for women. So, you will have around 9-10,000 calories to 'spend' over the week. Divide them as you wish between the five weekdays and the two weekend days. You might allow yourself 1,200 calories per weekday and 2,000 per weekend day.

It's up to you, whether to spread the indulgences through the week, or save them up for the weekend. You might choose to go on a 'light fast' (500-800 calories) on one or two of the weekdays, which would either allow for more treats at the weekend or speed up your weight loss.

If you don't go over your budget of calories, you should see your weight going down by 2-4 kilos per month. You will probably save your allowance of alcohol, cheese and/or chocolate for weekends, but you may decide to include a small quantity of one or other of them every day if you prefer.

At first, it may be hard to discipline yourself, but it will become easier as the weeks go by and your physical and psychological systems adjust to the regime you have chosen. When you start to see the results, enjoy it. Congratulate yourself on what you've achieved and encourage yourself to keep going. If it really doesn't suit you, feel free to let yourself off the leash from time to time, but you probably won't lose weight unless you keep your total weekly consumption within the guidelines. No problem. You may just need to spend a week or two extra on the reducing diet and put up with a small delay in hitting your target.

Missing a week is much better than giving up altogether. In fact, you may decide, say, after the first four weeks, that you need a week off, like the builders on the Great Wall. If so, no need to feel guilty. Just try it. See how it works for you.

It's best not to go totally crazy, otherwise you'll wipe out all those hard-won gains of the previous four weeks, but if there's some food that you've been thinking about and missing, treat yourself. Check what it does to your weight. Is it worth it? If so, why not make room for it in your regular reducing diet? Of course, you'll have to leave out something else to make room for it, but it's your choice.

It's always your choice, but try to let your True Self have the final say, rather than that Greedy Self.

'Do you think, because you are virtuous,
There shall be no more cakes and ale?'
Toby Belch, in the middle of a big night out, to the
wowser, Malvolio,
in *Twelfth Night*, Act 2, Scene 3,
by William Shakespeare

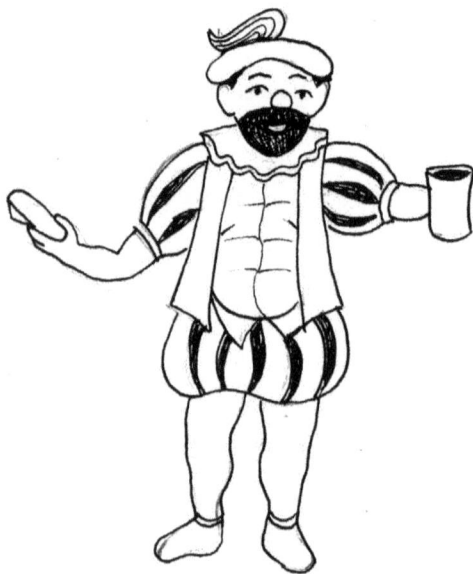

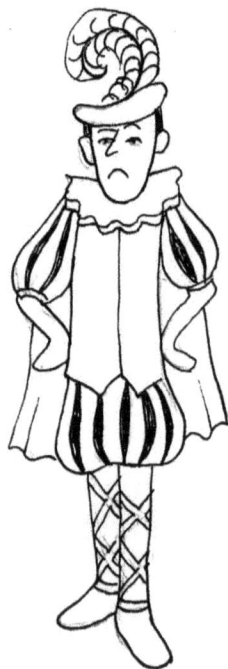

6

When can you stop?

The aim of this book is simple: it is to alert you to noble and admirable qualities you already possess, but which you may have come to doubt. You already have within you the strong willpower and determination you will need, to take charge of your everyday habits of eating, drinking and exercise and impose a beneficial discipline on yourself.

Your True Self really does know better than your Greedy Self what's best for you. You are perfectly capable of acting in accordance with your True Self's wishes and refusing the bribes, pleading, trickery and cajoling of your Greedy Self. Most of the time. And this is the most important point. No-one is perfect. No-one can succeed all of the time. You do possess powerful reserves of willpower and determination, but you're not Superman or Wonderwoman, are you? [If Superman or Wonderwoman happens to be reading this, I apologise: you are, of course, either Superman or Wonderwoman – but why are you reading about losing weight and lowering your cholesterol levels?]

Where was I? Yes, of course, there will be occasions when you succumb to temptation – maybe every day, probably every week. Your Greedy Self will seize on each instance to try and persuade you that, you see, you are weak-willed, you don't have the strength to resist, so why not give in altogether? Remind your Greedy Self about Winston Churchill. Tell it that it has had its fun and now your True Self is taking over again.

If your Greedy Self behaves itself, you may reward it with another treat next week, or next month, at a time of your choosing.

People who fall off a horse are advised to climb back on, as soon as they can. The same applies with weight loss diets. You are going to experience lapses in concentration or determination. You will give in to temptation. When you do, don't spoil the moment by feeling guilty. Savour it and enjoy it to the full. And then reassert control. Get back on the horse, which in your case is your pathway to greater health and fitness and a longer, happier life.

Rome wasn't built in a day and the amount of weight you want to shed won't be lost in a day, either. Once you've reached your target weight, you'll need a maintaining diet plan, to keep you there. In fact, you'll almost certainly need it, long before you reach your target weight. You'll find you break the rules of your reducing diet – probably sooner rather than later.

A maintaining diet plan that is perfect for YOU

It may be a special social occasion, a stressful day at work, fatigue, inattention, some particularly tempting delicacies on offer – any one of a huge number of events or circumstances can combine to throw us off our planned path. OK, feel guilty if it will help you to regroup, but don't decide you're worthless because you've failed: don't abandon your master plan. There will be many such lapses on your way to success: just enjoy them at the time and make sure they don't happen too often.

If your lapse is not too great or too gross, you may be able to mark the day down as a maintaining diet day – which is defined as a day in which you neither gain nor lose weight. Once you have reached your target weight, most of your days will be maintaining diet days. Having achieved your goal, you won't want to eat and drink everything in sight and have to start the process all over again, will you?

Your maintaining diet plan may not be radically different in character from your reducing diet plan. A little more food and drink, a little more variety, a few more occasions when you will allow yourself a drink, or some cheese or chocolate. Once you have got used to eating healthier, less calorific foods, you will probably find you don't want to go back to your old regime, full time. Your body will feel lighter and fitter and you'll want to keep it that way.

As with the reducing diet plan, you will need to work out a regime that suits your personal tastes and preferences, while keeping your weight within the parameters that you have decided to set. Once you have reached your target weight, you should set a figure about 3kg or 5-6lb above it, which you will declare to be 'the new fat' for you. When your bathroom scales tell you that you've put on that amount, as they undoubtedly will, at some time, you will simply need to revert to your reducing diet plan for a few days, or however long it takes to get back to your target weight. Don't put it off for too long or it may take a long time.

Of course, your lapse may be more substantial. As a lover of booze, cheese and chocolate who has been practising beneficial self-denial for a while, you may kick over the traces in a big way. As ever, make sure you enjoy every wicked mouthful. If inebriation is inevitable, lie back and enjoy it. Payback time will arrive all too soon. Such a day will not be on your maintaining diet plan, but your indulging diet plan. Yes, these are the days when you abandon yourself to the lusts of the belly, when your Greedy Self gets its way. They will be rare, so make the most of them.

An indulging diet plan that is perfect for YOU

While you are on the reducing diet plan, on the way to your target weight, you will not want to allow yourself too many indulgence days. The wine or beer, the cheeses, the chocolate will never have tasted so unbelievably delicious. If you have gone without them for a few days, the flavours and effects will be a revelation. One of the great rewards of abstinence is that it intensifies the pleasure, when you finally allow yourself to indulge again. So eat, drink and be merry, for tomorrow we diet again.

As with your reducing and maintaining diet plans, you will want to design your indulging diet plan with great care. Make sure you don't take on a massive load of calories unless they come in the form of a food or drink that you absolutely adore. Quality control is vital. Since the indulgences will be rarer than before, treat yourself to some very special delights.

They need not necessarily be expensive. After several weeks of severely limiting your carbohydrate intake, for example, a potato dish or a bowl of pasta or a plate of buttered toast may taste more exquisite and exotic than you can imagine. It will taste even better if you have earned it beforehand, so that both your True Self and your Greedy Self will agree that this is an approved indulgence.

Whether it is a planned and scheduled treat or a 'crash and burn' giving way to temptation, however, you will need to remember to call a halt when you have had enough. Don't 'pig out' unless every mouthful is a pleasure. There will come a reckoning. In the case of heavy carbs, you may need to take a substantial amount of extra exercise, the following day. As a rule of thumb, to work off a bowl of pasta, you will need to run well over 10km or the equivalent in your preferred form of exercise.

There is no free lunch, even on the Booze, Cheese and Chocolate Diet. But there will be some very fine lunches, and by creating and observing your three diet plans, reducing, maintaining and indulging, you will be able to ensure that such occasions are perfectly suited to your taste.

Don't ever eat or drink anything unless you really want it. Don't 'use up' food, to stop it going to waste: it will simply end up going to your waist. Don't eat to please others: if you don't really, really want to eat or drink something, after thinking about it, don't be afraid to refuse it, leave it or throw it away. Soon enough, you will come across something more to your taste, which you will then be able to enjoy with a clear conscience.

'I am a great eater of beef
And I believe that does harm to my wit.'
Sir Andrew Aguecheek, experiencing a rare moment of
self-awareness
in *Twelfth Night*, Act 1, Scene 1, by William Shakespeare

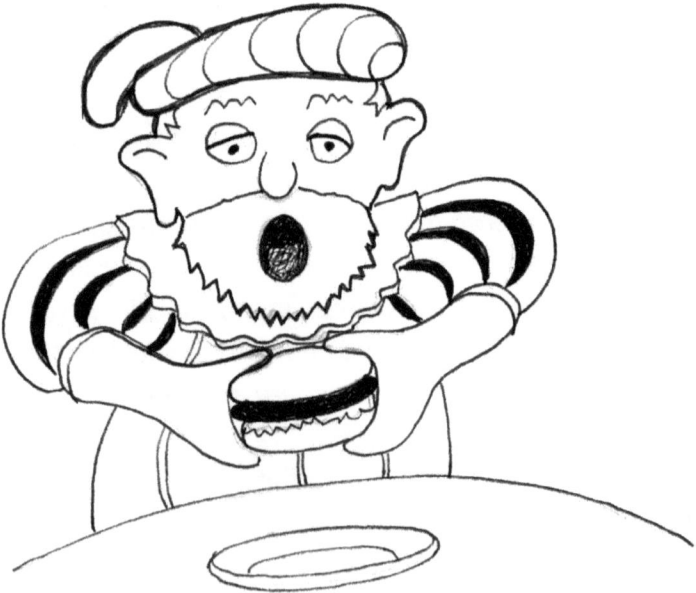

7

What's for Dinner?

If you really want to lose weight, it's helpful to understand exactly what effects various foods have on you. Think of it as arming your brain with knowledge that will help it to refuse the demands of your belly. You're the captain of this ship. It's your job to sail it safely around the world on your journey of a lifetime. You don't need heavy cargo, poor fuel or unfavourable wind – of any kind.

Your reducing diet will be lower in fats, for obvious reasons. It will also be low in carbohydrates (particularly the more refined and processed kinds) because, unless you burn them off with energetic exercise, they will simply trigger your body to make more fat. So, you will probably stop using bread, potatoes, rice and pasta to 'fill yourself up' as you may have done as a child. Your adult body needs a different grade of fuel.

Sugar, a simple carbohydrate, tends to undermine any reducing diet. You experience a brief energy hit from the sugar spike, but it will soon pass and leave you feeling hungry for more. Eating anything containing too much sugar or 'added sugar' will make your mission much more difficult. Nothing is completely banned in the Booze, Cheese and Chocolate Diet, but it's only common sense to find out which foods and beverages will help your aims and which will hinder them.

Certainly, you need protein, and it's essential to include some in your diet every day. You need a regular supply of protein to build and maintain your muscles. The idea is to lose weight without losing your strength. The average intake of protein required for adults up to the age of 70 is about 50-70gm for women and 60-100gm for men. Meat is a good source of protein but by no means the only one.

Vegetarians need to be especially careful that their diets include enough different sources of protein. Many pulses (the edible seeds of plants in the legume family, such as beans, peas, chickpeas and lentils) are high in protein, as are nuts, soy products, fish, eggs and almost all types of cheese. Most cheeses are also high in fat content – but some, like cottage cheese, manage to be both low-fat and high-protein. It's best to take a variety of protein-rich foods, because they help your body to create many different amino acids which you need, to stay healthy. Protein supplements in powdered form are useful for body-builders and athletes undertaking exceptional amounts of exercise, but for most people, a balanced, varied diet will supply all the protein that is required.

Food is fuel for your body.

You wouldn't try to run your car or truck on the wrong grade of fuel, just because it was a bit cheaper. Why would you economise on the fuel for your body? Bodies are much harder to repair and, despite the wonders of modern medicine and surgery, impossible to trade in and replace.

For a successful reducing diet plan, the trick is a delicate balancing act. Your aim will be to supply your body with all the nutrition it needs, to continue working at peak performance, while encouraging it to use up the stores of fat that it has laid by for that 'rainy day' when the habitual surplus stops arriving. If you can persuade your stomach that it has had enough fresh supplies delivered, while consuming only the daily allowance of calories you have set yourself, you will start to lose weight.

Most of the time, therefore, you will be eating foods that are low in calories but high in nutrition – lean meat, steamed or grilled fish, chicken breasts, fruit that is not too high in sugar and above all, fresh vegetables, either raw or cooked. You will also tend to choose more unprocessed or minimally processed whole foods (e.g. beans, seeds, nuts, whole grains, fresh fruit and vegetables) which are full of fibre, skin and antioxidants. These unprocessed foods are rich in nutrients, filling and slow to digest, so they will keep you going for longer and postpone those hunger pangs.

In the developed world, many of us have an irrational fear of hunger, which we use as an excuse for eating too much, too often or too soon. Fortunately, fainting from hunger is a very rare occurrence, but people convince themselves it might happen, if they miss a meal. So, we fill ourselves up with unnecessary, sugary foods before leaving home in the morning. Our bodies digest it swiftly and start craving for more of the same, often before the next meal is due.

We are creatures of habit and we create expectations in our bodies that are not always good for us. Your Greedy Self demands 'Feed me now!' – often loudly enough to drown out the wiser counsel of your True Self. A pang of hunger is not such a terrible pain – nothing, compared to a bad headache. It's a signal from your body that it is receiving less food than yesterday – which may be exactly what your True Self intends. Recent research by Dr Michael Mosley and others has proved that regular fasting can have highly beneficial effects on your metabolism. In particular, if it helps to break your habitual dependence on a regular intake of foods that you don't need, fasting can be a valuable tool in shaping the new you.

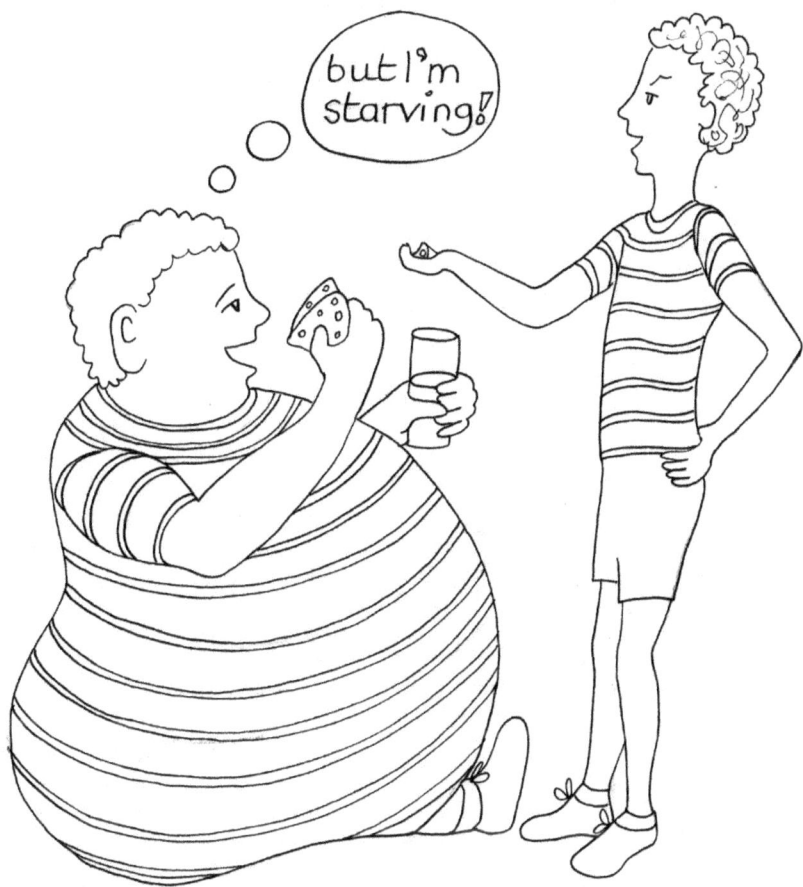

'My salad days,
When I was green in judgement, cold in blood'
Cleopatra, recalling the innocence and
naïvety of her youth
In *Antony & Cleopatra* Act 1, Scene 5,
by William Shakespeare

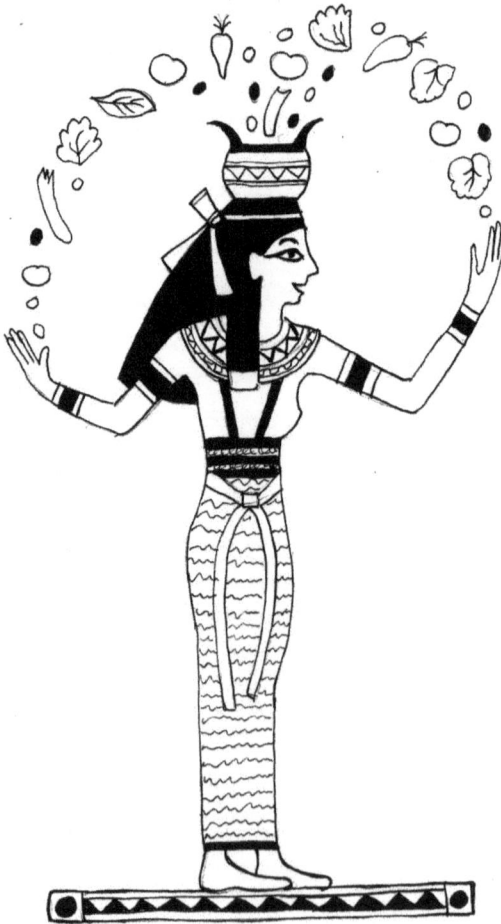

8

Will your friends be green with envy?

Nature has a way of colour-coding things, either to warn or to attract. Poisonous snakes and spiders are often garishly coloured; so are many deadly berries and fungi. The system isn't totally focused on human requirements, so it's not infallible, but it's a useful guide nevertheless.

Green is the universal signal of freshness, new growth, youth and springtime – when life begins all over again. Fruits that are green when unripe go yellow, orange and red to show they're ready for consumption. Many foods that are black, brown, grey or white are stale and past their best, unappetising or positively harmful. There are many exceptions to this rough rule, but it's a useful yardstick. Colour has always played a huge part in our selection of foods, and it still should.

Try an experiment with a banana: eat half of it and leave the other half intact, still inside the skin. Within an hour or two, the part of the skin that is empty will begin to go black, whereas the skin that still has fruit inside will remain bright yellow. This is the banana's way of signalling to birds and animals that ripe fruit is still available; it's trying to spread its seeds around the neighbourhood.

Even though that banana may have been picked weeks ago, it is still 'alive' enough to send out its signal. Ideally, most of the food you eat should retain its life force in this way. That's the power you're trying to harness, to support your own life. Canned or bottled foods are a fine tribute to human ingenuity and we wouldn't be without them – but, if you have a free choice, as most of us do, fresh is best.

If you're serious about losing weight, you'll learn to love the colour green – and all the other bright, fresh colours of the rainbow that say 'Eat me!' What you eat must give you pleasure, or you won't succeed in your aim. Much of your food will be yellow, red, orange and purple, as well as green, because of the precious antioxidants that lie just under the skins and in the cores and seeds. The best parts are often thrown away when foods are processed. Supermarkets trade nutrition for profit and a longer shelf-life. Bright colours often signify new life – the sort of life you can experience afresh if you shed several kilos of middle-aged fat.

Many vegetables have very few calories – so you can eat as much of them as you like. If you don't think you like vegies much, just find ways of preparing and serving them to make them more appetising.

A fresh approach to salads

Salads are much maligned: they often get a bad press, which they do not deserve. For your reducing diet plan to work, you need to find a way of making salad dishes hugely appealing to you. You need to channel some of the love and desire you may feel for booze, cheese and chocolate in the direction of the humble salad bowl. This will probably be easier than you expect.

The first conundrum to solve is when to eat it. If your typical idea of salad is of a bowl of limp lettuce leaves, drenched in a sharp, vinaigrette dressing, served immediately after a large helping of steak and chips, dismiss that image from your mind. Few people can raise much enthusiasm for such an offering after ingesting enough meat and fat to keep a family of four going for a week.

If you're serving your salad at dinnertime, make it the very first course. Hunger is the best sauce, so try to eat as little as you can get by on, through the day. That way, you will be ravenous for your salad, when it comes along. You'll be happy to eat quite a lot of it – and you can, with impunity, because most of the ingredients will have very few of those pesky calories. In addition, recent research indicates that eating your salad and vegetables right at the start of a meal can radically slow down your rate of glucose absorption, reducing inflammation and encouraging your body to store less fat.

Secondly, do everything you can to make your salad appealing to you and those with whom you share your meals. My favourite is basically an Everyday Greek Salad with infinite variations and additions, but it should contain several things that you find delicious. These may include:

Olives of whatever kind you prefer, big black Kalamata olives, tiny, intensely flavoured Ligurian ones, green olives stuffed with chilli or garlic – the choice is yours.

Avocado, preferably ripe and fresh, divided into tiny pieces with a teaspoon. It doesn't matter if it melts and blends in with the dressing – it will still taste delicious.

Tomatoes, probably some sundried ones for extra flavour but plenty of fresh, ripe ones, cut up if they are big and just halved if they are small – but cut into them, to release the juicy aromas and taste! Add a little salt before mixing them with the other ingredients.

Cucumbers, preferably the small 'Lebanese' variety, for flavour and digestibility, sliced or diced to mix with the rest.

Feta cheese, if you like it, or Cottage cheese, which has less flavour but considerably fewer calories. The cheese is there principally to enhance the dressing, so cut it small. A word of warning: the Feta and avocado both have a few calories, so use one or the other or a little of each.

Red Onion, much sweeter than other varieties, chopped very small and mixed through the salad.

Garlic, if you like it, a whole clove or even two, crushed and mixed in.

Capsicum of whatever colour appeals, also chopped small, but still large enough to taste each piece.

Celery, young, chopped small, not too much.

Radishes, chopped, to add a bit of zest and pep.

Radicchio, Italian 'red lettuce' a very distinctive, slightly bitter flavour.

Watercress, peppery and well worth the time it takes to break the fresh, tender leaves off from the stems, which can be tough to chew.

Rocket, 'ruccola', another flavoursome Italian miracle.

Spinach leaves, young, fresh and not too big.

Lettuce, if you can find a variety that tastes of something more interesting than water. We humans have something in common with lettuce: we, too, are over 90% water – but we usually have more flavour.

Vegetables, cooked and added cold – beans, peas, sweet corn, asparagus, broccolini and many more. It's your call.

Sprouted seeds of all kinds are highly nutritious and add variety.

Fresh Herbs, Mint, Tarragon, Basil, any you like, but preferably not those dried herbs that have been sitting in a glass jar in your larder for the past ten years: any flavour they had will have evaporated long ago.

Chilli, fresh and chopped into tiny pieces, or dry flakes.

Nuts and Dry Seeds, not too many nuts, because the calories can sneak up on you, but a few pine nuts, pistachios, pepitas (husked pumpkin seeds), sunflower seeds, sesame seeds, linseeds, chia seeds, etc., scattered over the top of the bowl as a final flourish.

Olive Oil only, for a true Greek salad, the best quality you can afford, Extra Virgin (a confusing concept), preferably the first, cold press.

Sesame Seed Oil for added flavour, or other exotic oils.

Soy Sauce or Truffle Salt, tastier than plain salt.

If you adapt the ingredients to suit your own likes and dislikes, this kind of salad can easily become the main meal of your day, and one you will look forward to and relish. It's really good for you and if you're careful with the high-calorie items, such as nuts and oils, the weight will fall off you in a way that may be just as satisfying as your everyday salad.

For a 'proper dinner', you also need a portion of protein. This might take the form of grilled fish or chicken or a small amount of lean meat, which you might like to serve with an additional cooked vegetable or two – but try not to add too much in the way of oils, sauce or butter as garnish. Alternatively, you might add some flakes of cold salmon or ocean trout, anchovies, prawns or even eggs to the salad and make it a single course meal. See later notes if you're trying to cut down on cholesterol.

Crunchy Salads

I prefer to serve a crunchy salad separately, because it's satisfying to have a good chew, but not all the way through the meal. Crunchy salads can be made with grated raw carrots and beetroots, finely chopped red cabbage and other vegetables and enlivened with a few raisins and seeds. Mayonnaise enhances it enormously but can easily add more calories than you need, so go easy on it. Cottage cheese is a good low-calorie alternative if you want something to moisten the mixture.

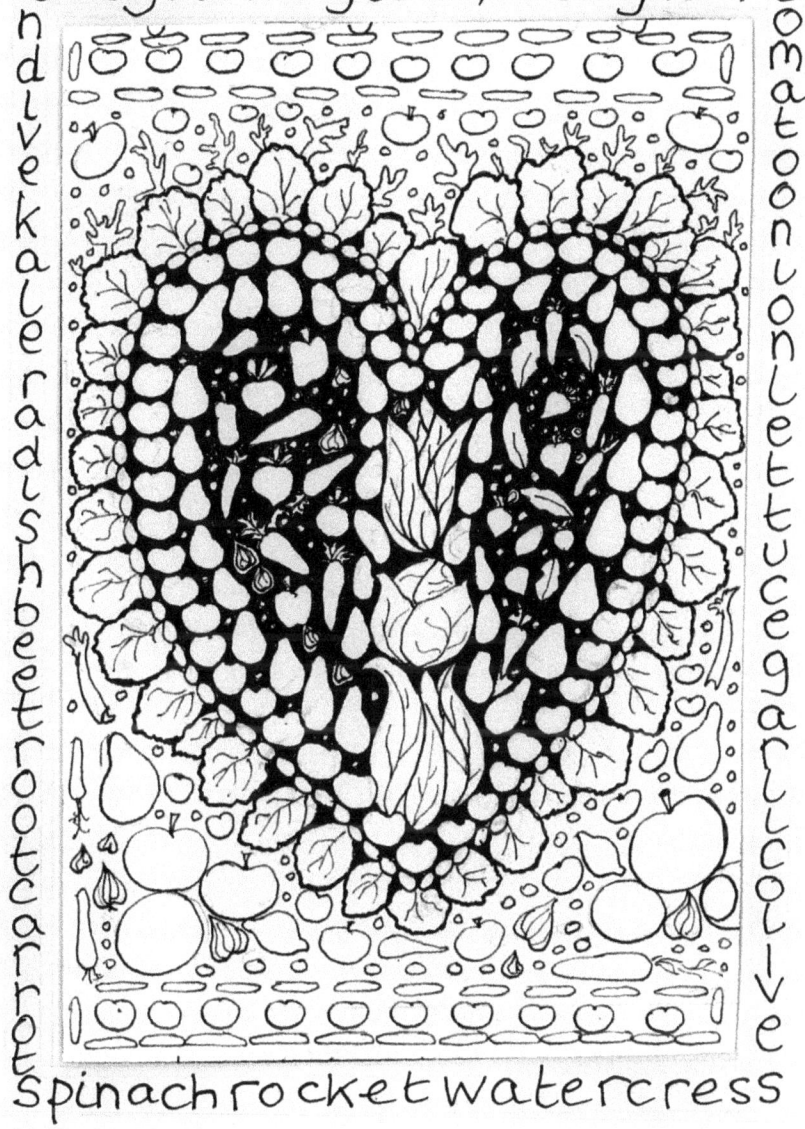

eatyourwaytoahealthyheart

endivekaleradishbeetrootcarrot

tomatoonionlettucegarlicolive

spinachrocketwatercress

53

'Drink, sir, is a great provoker of three things:
Nose painting, sleep and urine.
Lechery, sir, it provokes and unprovokes:
It provokes the desire but takes away the performance.'
The Porter at Macbeth's castle, roused from sleep by
latecomers in *Macbeth*, Act 2, Scene 3,
by William Shakespeare

'A man cannot make him laugh,
But that's no marvel: he drinks no wine!'
Sir John Falstaff, giving his opinion of non-drinkers
in *King Henry IV, Part Two*, Act 2, Scene 4,
by William Shakespeare

'Good wine, sir, is a familiar creature
If it be well used. Exclaim no more against it.'
The villainous Iago, telling Cassio not to blame
drink for his downfall in *Othello*, Act 2, Scene 3,
by William Shakespeare

'Come, gentleman, I hope we shall drink down
All unkindness.'
Slender, at the start of a bender in *The Merry Wives
of Windsor*, Act 1, Scene 1, by William Shakespeare

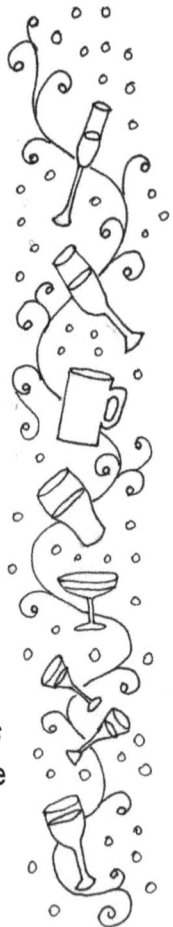

'Why, sir, for my part, I say the gentleman
Had drunk himself out of his five senses!'
Bardolph, calling Slender too drunk to remember the
bender in *The Merry Wives of Windsor*, Act 1, Scene 1,
by William Shakespeare

9

Drinking your health

Shakespeare, eat your heart out. Peter Fitzsimons, a former Wallaby and currently one of the most readable columnists on *The Sydney Morning Herald*, takes the cakes and ale for coming up with the definitive remark on alcohol consumption:

'It's a better night with it, but a better life without it.'

The most hardened drinkers would find it difficult to disagree with that brutally honest assessment. On the other hand, another eloquent Aussie, the late, lamented Clive James (echoing WC Fields), observed:

'We can, none of us, hope to get out of this world alive.'

Are we, therefore, going to drink ourselves to death? That would be a terrible waste of the lithe and lissom new figure we are about to attain. So let's admit that we're probably on a journey towards giving up alcohol, not necessarily obsessively, perhaps not even completely, certainly not now, but at some unspecified time in the future, let's say, before we reach what we would be prepared to call 'Old Age'.

Few of the very ancient people I know still imbibe with the enthusiastic fervour of their youth. So it's really just a question of when, this side of our encounter with the Grim Reaper, we are going to 'sign the pledge' and abjure the demon drink forever.

I suggest not yet. Not when you are about to embark on the Booze, Cheese and Chocolate Diet, which promises to provide you with the best of all worlds, the ability to continue enjoying the most pleasurable indulgences while being the proud possessor of a physique that would not look out of place in – well, in your own bathroom mirror, for a very good start.

One of the problems is that alcohol is a food – which means it contains calories, and is therefore, to a degree, fattening – but it is not, by common consent, a whole food, or indeed an entirely wholesome food.

It can be enjoyed in moderation – in the Booze, Cheese and Chocolate Diet, as in life. Alcohol, in all its many wondrous guises and disguises, is a source of much fun and pleasure, but it has a sharp sting in its tail.

How much is too much?

If not handled wisely and with respect, alcohol can do us harm, in many ways. It can make us look and sound like idiots. It can cost us our driving licences. It can lay us open to divorce and many deeply unpleasant, degenerative diseases. It can even make us drop dead, drunk in a ditch.

The thoughtful drinker faces these challenges squarely, head on, man to man. (It has to be a man, doesn't it?) He raises his glass to them and pronounces:

'Cheers, mate. You've got a fair point. But you're a long time dead. It's not going to happen just yet, is it?'

Maybe this only goes to show that deep drinkers are not necessarily deep thinkers. Alcohol can be as deceiving as our Greedy Self. When they both work together, they can run rings around our True Self. You are going to allow your True Self to decide what you eat and how much: well, it is even more important to make sure it is your True Self that decides what you drink – how much and how often.

If you feel you are incapable of drinking in moderation, the wisest decision is not to drink at all, or only on very rare occasions. Portion control is essential. Any alcohol you allow yourself means eating less food, because these calories count, as well. If you're content with a small glass of wine or spirits every day, you could conceivably incorporate it into your reducing diet, at a cost of calories in other forms.

If you prefer to have two or three glasses at a sitting, you will need to ration your drinking to two evenings a week, probably at the weekends. If you like to drink a whole bottle of wine by yourself, you will be drinking only once a week – and probably sleeping by yourself, as well.

Just as with your intake of food, it's essential to have a clear understanding of how many calories there are in each drink you take – because they will make their way to exactly the same places as the calories in your food. You can afford to eat more or drink more, within your self-imposed budget of calories, and still achieve your target weight – but not both. The good news, if you like a drink, is that it is not incompatible with your weight loss program. You simply need to make an informed decision on how much you are going to allow yourself – and adjust your three diet plans, reducing, maintaining and indulging, in accordance with that plan – and then stick to it! (Maybe the hardest part)

Counting the cost in calories

A 750ml bottle of wine contains about 600 calories, so each 150ml (5oz) glass has 120 calories or so, consisting of less than 1g of protein, 4g of carbohydrates and 15g of alcohol. Sweeter wines have more calories and so do wines with more alcohol. Watch the quantities: restaurants serve 125ml but you could be pouring yourself up to 250ml at home.

If you prefer spirits, the news is not so bad. A 25ml measure of most spirits contains a shade over 50 calories, which rises to 80 for sweet liqueurs. If you take tonic with your gin, or any other mixer, you'll need to allow for those calories as well, but even on your reducing diet plan, you can probably afford to have either a small drink each night or half a dozen drinks at the weekend. But are you only pouring yourself 25ml?

For beer drinkers, life is tougher. The term 'beer gut' is not a misnomer. A 375ml glass of most beers comes in somewhere between 130 and 150 calories, depending on sugar content and ABV. That's about the equivalent of a Mars Bar (136 calories). The very strong, unbelievably delicious Belgian beers with ABVs above 10% can have twice as many calories as the ordinary stuff. It's probably a good thing you can't drink too many of them without falling over. The unavoidable conclusion is that you are unlikely to lose weight unless you restrict your beer drinking to weekends – and then monitor the quantities closely. You probably don't need me to remind you that, once you've started drinking, it's terribly easy to drink more than you intended – of beer or anything else.

But, drinkers all, be of good cheer! (Drinkers usually are.) Things could be worse. Your favourite tipple, be it a sparkling Prosecco, a mellow Malbec, an expensive Espresso Martini or a head-banging Chimay Blue, is less dangerous to your health than other common addictions, chosen or suffered by millions of people, around the world.

Be thankful you're not a fast food fanatic. If you were, you'd blow your daily calorie budget quicker than you could order an average hamburger with large fries and a milkshake to wash it down.

You could probably afford to consume that lot, without exceeding your daily budget of calories, but you wouldn't be eating or drinking anything else that day – and you would have set several weeks' allowance of viscous cholesterol and triglycerides circulating greasily around your delicate veins and arteries, looking for something to block. Cheers!

'I will make an end of my dinner:
There's pippins and cheese to come!'
Sir Hugh Evans, clearly a cheese-lover,
in *The Merry Wives of Windsor*, Act 1, Scene 2,
by William Shakespeare

'I had rather live
With garlic and cheese in a windmill, far,
Than feed on cakes and have him talk to me
In any summerhouse in Christendom.'
Harry Hotspur, no fan of cheese, garlic or his father-in-law's advice,
in *King Henry IV, Part One*, Act 3, Scene 1,
by William Shakespeare

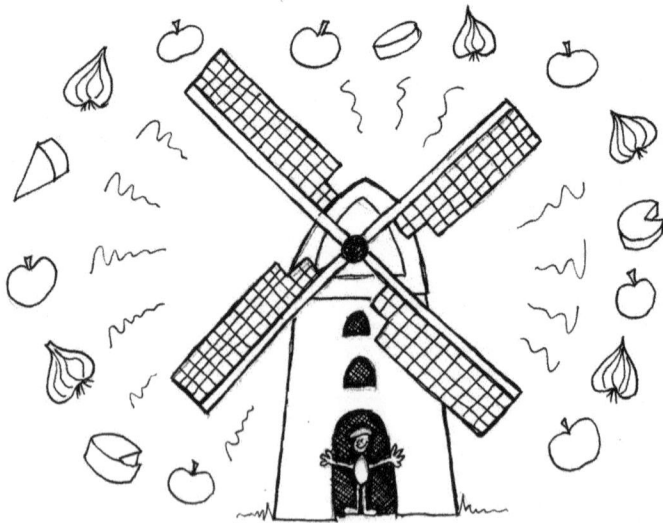

10

Do you have a friend in cheeses?

If God hadn't invented cheeses, we'd never have needed to invent God. Cheese is the strongest evidence around of a mysterious, higher power. It guides our destinies and leads us gently to greener pastures, where strange, placid beasts quietly ruminate. Their milk is magically transformed into an infinite variety of spellbinding flavours. If there is a Heaven, there may not be angels, but there will certainly be cheese.

Wise Ulysees, in Homer's *Odyssey*, conceived an original way of resisting temptation, when his ship sailed past the island of the Sirens. Their seductive songs so enraptured passing sailors that they hurled themselves into the raging seas, desperate to reach the enchantresses, and drowned. Ulysees made his crew block their ears with beeswax and told them to lash him firmly to the mast for the passage past the island. He ordered them to ignore any pleas he might later make to be set free. Whatever happened, they must leave him tightly bound until their ship was safely out of earshot of the Sirens.

This story has fascinated people ever since. It still speaks to us, across thirty centuries, because it understands the dynamic between pleasure and temptation.

Why did Ulysees not block his own ears with beeswax? Because he wanted to experience the exquisite delight of hearing the Sirens' songs, without paying the customary penalty. Cheese-lovers will see in it at once a metaphor for their own weakness – which they may legitimately choose to regard as a strength!

Cheese goes back a long way. It was invented long before writing and reading. One or more of our ancestors probably tried to store some milk in an animal's stomach, where the enzyme rennet naturally occurs, and found the milk was first curdled and then preserved. They found that adding other ingredients, like herbs and spices, food acids and wood smoke, developed an incredible range of different flavours.

Homer knew a lot about cheese. His fearsome, one-eyed Cyclops, Polyphemus, kept flocks of sheep and goats and brought them into the vast cave where he lived, to milk them, every night. Half of the milk, he drank with his dinner. The other half, he made into cheese and stored in the cave. When Ulysees and his men helped themselves to his cheeses, he imprisoned them and ate some of them alive – clearly an over-reaction – but he was a cheese-maker, so he can't have been all bad.

Learn from Ulysees and the Sirens

There is an important lesson here for all cheese-lovers. If you loosen the shackles and just set yourself free to behave like a glutton, every time you sail past a cheeseboard, the consequences will be dire. Cheese is one of the wonders of the culinary world, but it's not worth dying for

You can indulge your senses to the full, savour the siren songs of all the cheeses you love and still reach safe harbour, but only if you approach the problem in a highly intelligent, discriminating and determined way. Like Ulysees, your aim must be to extract maximum enjoyment, with minimum punishment. You are going to follow this approach with your diet as a whole: simply apply the same principles to your cheese-eating.

Since you are going to limit your total consumption of cheese, in the interest of controlling your weight and waistline, make sure the cheese you do eat is excellent. It would be absurd to waste your allowance of cheese-calories on poor quality, processed cheeses.

Find a cheese merchant offering a wide variety of first class supplies. S/he may run a market stall or an expensive boutique, but is unlikely to be found in a supermarket. S/he will know and care about cheeses and be generous with advice about them. The best cheese merchants are always happy to offer tastes of their wares: words can only go so far.

A wine merchant once told me to 'Buy with apples, sell with cheese'. What he meant was, if you take small bites of apple, between tasting wines, it will refresh your palate and help you to assess the next one. On the other hand, he advised, free cheese makes any wine taste good!

Buy your cheese in small quantities – for two reasons: first, because, if you have a lot of cheese in the house, you will eat more than you intend, and secondly, because many cheeses decline quite swiftly and you will want to enjoy them at their peak. If you keep cheese in a refrigerator, be careful to restore it to room temperature well before you consume it. Serving or eating cheese too cold is a terrible waste.

Cut your cheese thinly, rather than in big chunks. The aim is to extract the maximum flavour: a greater surface area gives you more chance to taste it. Don't swallow it quickly, just because you're greedy for the next piece: that would be counter-productive. Experience the way the various flavours develop in your mouth – much as you might with a special wine. Enjoy the moment and make it last.

What else goes with cheese?

Think carefully about what you combine with your cheese. With a full-flavoured cheese, many people tend to take a larger quantity of bread or crackers and butter, to absorb some of the strength or sharpness. Why not cut out the supporting cast and concentrate on the star of the show? You'll achieve the same taste experience with less cheese – so you can have some more, later.

When cooked, cheese can be a great enhancement to pasta and potato dishes – but be careful that you're not eating a lot of carbohydrates you don't really want. If you wouldn't eat the pasta or potatoes without the cheese, why not eat the cheese by itself, to help cut back on the carbs?

French President Charles de Gaulle once asked rhetorically, 'How can you possibly govern a nation that has 246 cheeses?' The gourmet who first proposed a low carbohydrate diet, Brillat-Savarin, after whom one of those cheeses is named, observed: 'A dinner without cheese is like a beautiful woman with only one eye.'

France has developed many of the finest cheeses, but doesn't have a monopoly: there are over a thousand different kinds, worldwide – far too many for one person to taste in a lifetime, but don't let that stop you trying. It's tempting to stick with a few old favourites, but fortune favours the brave: it's exciting to experiment and discover a new taste-treasure. All the more reason to buy cheeses in small quantities. And new ones!

An infinite variety

Cheese is basically the curdled, concentrated milk of cows, sheep, goats and buffaloes, that has been preserved. Experts differ, but it can be divided into five categories – Fresh, Soft, Washed Rind, Hard and Blue.

Fresh cheeses include Cottage cheese, Feta and Mozzarella. They don't last as long as more complex cheeses and they tend to be lighter on both calories and flavour. Cottage cheese, in particular, is a boon for calorie-conscious consumers and can be very effectively used as a substitute for Feta in your Everyday Greek Salad.

Soft cheeses include Brie and Camembert and for them, ripeness is all. The riper they are, the softer, creamier, tastier and more mobile they will become. If you can, hold off until they seem to crawl across the plate towards you, whispering 'Eat me!' The rewards will be worth waiting for.

Washed Rind cheeses like Époisses, Tallegio or Stinking Bishop, whose rind often shows signs of mould, have been soaked and ripened with bacteria from a wide variety of additives, and generally have fuller, richer flavours. They offer the widest range for fresh experiments. Be brave!

Hard cheeses are made by cutting and compressing the curds to reduce moisture and then storing them for months or years, to develop complex flavours. Cheddar and Parmigiano-Reggiano are full-flavoured pressed cheeses. Edam and Gouda are also hard cheeses, but they taste much milder because their curds have been rinsed in warm water.

Blue cheeses, like Stilton, Gorgonzola and Roquefort usually have the strongest flavours of all. They are often referred to as an acquired taste, but be warned: once you have acquired a taste for them, you will have it for life. They are usually injected with gut-friendly bacteria, so that the process of fermentation takes place inside the rind. The strong flavours mean that you don't need to eat huge quantities. A little blue cheese can transform a simple dish like Mushroom Soup.

Can you claim that cheese is good for you?

Well, a good soft cheese has valuable probiotics for gut health. Cheeses do contain useful amounts of protein and calcium but also loads of salt and saturated fats. These will raise your levels of LDL cholesterol (yes, the dangerous kind) and increase your risk of cardiovascular disease. Non-Vegan vegetarians can claim they need the protein, but that excuse is not available to carnivores.

Sadly, cheese is pretty well indefensible on nutritional grounds – but there is nothing else quite like it. Let's be honest: it's a dangerous indulgence. If you can resist it, you probably should. It will leave room in your indulgence diet for other, less harmful treats.

If you can't resist it, you're not alone. The best advice is to emulate wise Ulysses and enjoy being tempted without dying for it. Don't tuck into cheese every day: save it for special occasions. If you love cheese, don't try to give it up altogether, because you probably won't succeed. Just eat it mindfully, joyfully and in moderation.

'I love long life better than figs!'
Charmian, on being told by a Soothsayer that she will
outlive Cleopatra
in *Antony & Cleopatra*, Act 1, Scene 2,
by William Shakespeare

'Things sweet to taste prove in digestion sour.'
John of Gaunt, on learning that his son is to be banished
for six years
in *King Richard II*, Act 1, Scene 3,
by William Shakespeare

'What use are cartridges in battle?
I always carry chocolate instead!'
by George Bernard Shaw, in *Arms and the Man*, Act 1.

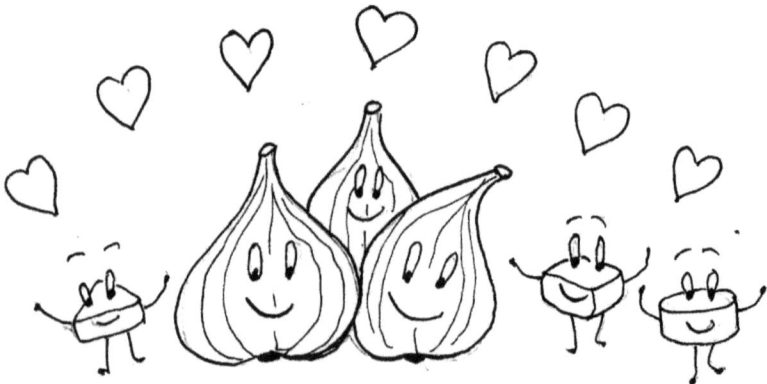

11

How sweet are sweets?
The joy of tantric chocolate

Sadly for the Bard of Avon and for ourselves, chocolate reached Britain many years after Will Shakespeare left the stage. Otherwise, he would have had heaps to say about it. How disappointing, that the greatest master of the English language never experienced that pleasure, and so never had his eloquence and superlatives truly stretched to the limit.

Sugar is a highly processed, simple carbohydrate and the deadliest enemy of all weight loss regimes. If you can drastically reduce the sugar in your diet, you will do yourself a huge favour and be well on the way to reaching your target weight surprisingly soon. But if you reckon chocolate is a special case, I'm with you all the way.

The problem is that most chocolate is roughly half sugar. You wouldn't dream of taking a teaspoon of sugar by itself, but you might easily eat a 100-gram (3.5oz) bar containing over a dozen teaspoons of sugar.

In a couple of minutes, you would consume more than the maximum daily allowance of added sugar recommended by the American Health Association. This is nine teaspoons (37.5g) for men and six (25g) for women. So, you couldn't allow yourself any more sugar for the rest of that day and most of the next.

In addition, that rapidly vanishing bar of chocolate will have supplied you with between 500 and 550 calories, almost as much as a whole bottle of wine or a decent portion of delicious cheese, and close to two-thirds of your total food ration for the day, on your reducing diet plan.

There is a solution, but it will involve a revolution in the way you eat chocolate. Ask yourself why you are eating it in the first place: it's not to pile on the calories or suck up the sugar, is it? It's for the flavour. And you can enjoy the taste of chocolate without eating a whole bar of it.

The most miraculous quality of chocolate is that it melts in your mouth – quite literally. It is designed to return to its liquid state at precisely your body temperature. So think hard, the next time you eat chocolate. Concentrate. It may take a while to change the habit of a lifetime, but you can do it. Don't take huge mouthfuls: you will find tiny quantities of chocolate will impart just as much flavour, if you give them time to do their work. Don't swallow it straight down: let it melt and work its magic.

A fresh approach to chocolate

First of all, try to choose chocolate with less sugar. Some brands of good quality, dark chocolate have 70%, 85%, even 95% cocoa, meaning much less sugar and a much more intense chocolate flavour. If you don't like it at first, persevere. It's probably the sugar your body is craving and it may take a while to adjust to the more chocolatey taste. It's very rich.

Say your 100-gram bar of chocolate comes in 10 squares, five rows of two. Break off two squares and put one back or give it to your partner, preparing it in the same way as your own portion. Cut each square into four, six or even a dozen tiny pieces. Eat one piece – by which I mean – put it in your mouth. Don't talk. You'll have plenty of time for talking later.

Right now, you are doing something very important: you are eating chocolate – and maybe tasting it fully for the first time. Don't bite into it. Let it melt. See how the flavour fills your mouth. Notice how it lasts. Only when it has completely melted, swallow it and notice how long the taste lingers on. When it has finally gone, have another piece. And another.

You'll spend 20-30 minutes with your mouth full of chocolate and you will taste every last morsel. If you find the pieces you have cut are too small at first to achieve the effect I have described, take two at a time. If you persevere and eat it mindfully and slowly, a tiny piece will be quite enough. Don't forget to let it melt in your mouth: that is the true wonder of chocolate. Try not to swallow it too soon: once you do that, the taste will start to fade away.

I apologise if this seems like trying to teach my grandmother to suck eggs, but humour me. Just try it, as an experiment. If you succeed, your chocolate-eating experience will last for up to half-an-hour and it will probably be quite enough to satisfy your hunger for chocolate for the whole day. If not, repeat the process.

Your one small square of chocolate (10g) will amount to only 50-60 calories, a small percentage of your daily allowance. Even so, you will have eaten the equivalent of a teaspoon of sugar, but very much less than if you'd chomped through a commercial chocolate bar in a couple of minutes, without really enjoying it.

On these figures, you don't have to save up your chocolate ration for your few days on an indulging diet plan: you could easily include this amount in your maintaining and even your reducing diet plans, as a regular after-dinner treat, perhaps with some fruit or coffee, for dessert.

Food of the gods

Chocolate has been consumed in Central and Southern America for close on 4,000 years, but in very different forms to those we enjoy today. The Aztecs liked a bitter drink made from fermented cocoa beans, called xocoatl in their language. This was probably the origin of most of the common words for chocolate in European languages – but the Latin name of the cocoa tree is more revealing: theobroma cacao, the food of the gods. In Aztec and Mayan communities, the beans were used as currency. You could buy a tamale snack for one bean, a ripe avocado for three or a live turkey for 100 beans.

The liquid chocolate was usually reserved for special occasions, which included human sacrifices. Even the victims were allowed a cup or two, to raise their spirits for the coming ordeal. The Aztec King Montezuma welcomed the Spanish explorer, Hernando Cortes, and his men with a great feast and served the ceremonial drink. The visitors were distinctly unimpressed and wrote scathing assessments in their journals. Nevertheless, they had the sense to take some of the precious beans back with them to Europe. There, some bright spark mixed the ground beans with honey or cane sugar, which made it much more palatable.

In the 1600s, rumours of the medicinal or aphrodisiac properties of chocolate added to its allure. Chocolate houses sprang up in wealthier districts, all over Europe. However, it was still an exclusive preserve of the privileged classes. It was only when the Industrial Revolution created new manufacturing processes that the new delicacy could be produced cheaply enough and in sufficient quantities for the 'huddled masses' to get their share.

In the nineteenth century, several of the names still associated with chocolate today, (Van Houten in the Netherlands, Nestlé in Switzerland, Fry, Rowntree and Cadbury in the UK and Hershey in the USA), developed complicated processes for refining ground cocoa solids into cocoa butter and blending them both with added milk and sugar to make solid and mouldable products. Mass production of chocolate was soon followed by mass addiction to it.

Joshua Fry's company showed a keen awareness of the mood-lifting power of their product: one of their popular chocolate bars was called Five Boys. Every bar was moulded with the faces of five youngsters at different stages of chocoholism. They were labelled: Desperation, Pacification, Expectation, Acclamation and Realisation – it's Fry's!

'As men do walk a mile, women should talk an hour,
After supper. It is their exercise.'
by Francis Beaumont and John Fletcher (1579-1625),
politically incorrect contemporaries of Shakespeare,
in their play *Philaster*, Act 2, Scene 4.

'Better to hunt in fields, for health unbought,
Than fee the doctor for a nauseous draught.
The wise, for cure, on exercise depend;
God never made his work for man to mend.'
by John Dryden (1631-1700) in his *Epistle to a Kinsman*,
John Driden of Chesterton

'Reading is to the mind what exercise is to the body.'
by Sir Richard Steele (1672-1729) in *The Tatler*,
which he founded.

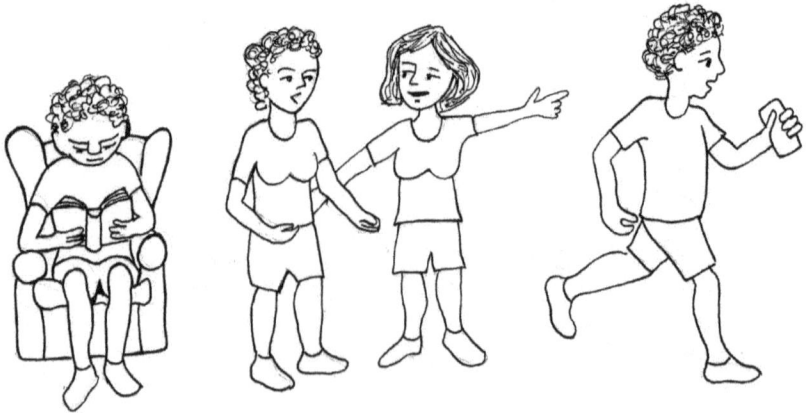

12

You're eating less,
but are you moving more?

There are, you will remember, two parts to the weight loss regime of the Booze, Cheese and Chocolate Diet, and neither part can achieve the result you desire without the other. Our mission statement could hardly be simpler – 'Eat Less, Move More' – and yet it is surprisingly easy, with all the other things we have to do and think about, to let one or the other slip for a day or two – or three or four, and in no time, the days have become weeks, and our project is in tatters.

If this happens to you – and it may, unless you are much more self-disciplined than most people who enjoy booze, cheese and chocolate – don't beat yourself up about your past failures, because there is absolutely nothing you can do anything about them. Just make sure you re-establish your regular routine as soon as you possibly can.

As with what you choose to eat and drink, the type and amount of exercise you take is entirely up to you – but you will need to manage at least four or five days, each week. You may decide to start slowly and build up gradually: that depends on your age, present level of fitness and whether you are already in the habit of exercising regularly. Remember that every step you take, every flight of stairs you elect to climb, every weight you lift is burning off calories and helping you to your goal.

Like Winston Churchill, you have 'nothing to offer but blood, toil, tears and sweat', as he told the House of Commons in his first speech to Parliament as Prime Minister in May 1940. You will certainly hope to circulate your blood, rather than shedding it, but it will play its part.

An equally memorable but anonymous saying goes: 'Horses sweat; gentlemen perspire; and ladies merely feel the heat.' Well, on the Booze Cheese and Chocolate Diet, we take it up a notch: gentlemen are expected to behave like horses and ladies like gentlemen.

It's important to choose a form of exercise that you will find at least congenial, and hopefully enjoyable. Your True Self is going to have to work out some way of persuading your Greedy Self (in this area, better known as your Lazy Self, but essentially the same) to hit the road, or the cycle track, or the gym, or the pool, or the river, or the exercise bike at home, or the tennis court, or the football field – on a regular basis, come rain or shine, come long days at work or a busy social diary.

Don't just do it: enjoy it

The pleasure principle is fundamental to the Booze, Cheese and Chocolate Diet. People who choose to lose weight in this way want to have their cake and eat it – literally! You want to enjoy the pleasures of life as well as improving your levels of health and fitness.

So you need to find a way of taking regular exercise that you'll enjoy. Otherwise you won't exercise as often as you should – and you'll have to compensate for that by eating and drinking even less.

The aim is to get your heart beating at exercise level for at least 20-30 minutes every day – or 4-5 days a week if you want to give yourself some leeway for rainy days or busy days when you just can't fit it into your schedule. The test of any activity is whether you work up a sweat – so energetic gardening might qualify as exercise for one day but a round of golf may not be lively enough, unless you're going to zip around the fairways like a young gazelle.

One of the secrets is to find the right time of day for exercise – the time that suits you. Maybe it's the early morning: try getting up earlier and setting aside some exercise time before you start on everything else. That way, for the rest of the day, you can pat yourself on the back, in the knowledge that, whatever else happens, you've nailed your exercise quota. It may help to stiffen your resolve to stick to your diet plan for the rest of the day, as well.

One obvious way of scheduling regular exercise is to join a gym – but joining isn't enough. You also need to motivate yourself to go there and do the work. Before you sign up, try it out. Make sure it's the right choice for you. If you were to sign up and then change your mind, the setback might undermine your determination to keep to your diet plan. Success breeds success, it's true, but on the other hand, failure in one area often leads to failure in another: only choose the gym option if you're sure it's going to galvanise you into action.

If you do sign up for a gym membership, take full advantage of the professional help on offer. Talk to a personal trainer, explain what your aim is, and get some help to design just the right program to keep you interested. Don't push yourself too hard at the beginning: build up gradually, so that you don't allow any stiffness or injuries to slow your progress. As the weeks go by, you'll see some pleasing improvement in your strength, muscle tone and overall fitness. If you get it right, you'll start looking forward to exercise, rather than seeing it as an obligation.

Anima (mens) sana in corpore sano

It was the Roman poet, Juvenal, who first pointed out the mutually beneficial effects of having both a healthy mind and a healthy body. He argued that these were greater blessings than the conventional markers of success, such as wealth and power, having people listen when you speak and producing many children. He also admitted that, however sound his advice and recommendations might be, only his readers could give these gifts to themselves. What a wise old bird Juvenal was!

The true value of exercise may not be apparent to you until you have managed to make it an inseparable part of your daily life. Of course, if you are limiting your intake of calories, it is a good idea to burn some off, at the same time – but the reasons for taking regular exercise go much deeper than that. If you persevere, you will find many other benefits, which you may not have considered.

One benefit is the way in which your central nervous system and your pituitary gland will start to release endorphins. The term originates from 'endogenous morphine', substances which counteract pain in the body and simulate euphoric pleasure. If you are not in the habit of exercising regularly, you may have to work your way through a number of pain barriers, before you can achieve this desirable state, but rest assured, it does exist and it will make you surprisingly keen for even more exercise.

Beyond the zone of pleasure, however, lie even greater benefits: the sharpness of your mind, your ability to process information and to continue working at optimum level, your moods and your overall sense of wellbeing will all be enhanced – as a direct result of knowing that your body is working more easily and more efficiently. By increasing your neuroplasticity, you will counteract or delay the onset of various neurodegenerative diseases, like Alzheimer's, Parkinson's and others.

The balance between positive and negative views will start to swing in your favour: the challenges you face will be less daunting and you will be less fearful of failure, because you will have a stronger belief in your ability to determine your own future and the nature of your environment.

If you don't believe me, just give it a try. Try to prove me wrong, if you like. Just to be clear, however, I'm not promising an easy, overnight transformation. I'm saying that, if you dedicate yourself for 3-4 months to a routine of regular exercise, you will succeed, not only in your weight loss program, but in many other areas of your life, as well.

'It takes all the running you can do,
to stay in the same place.
If you want to get somewhere else,
you must run at least twice as fast as that!'
by Lewis Carroll in *Through the Looking Glass*

'Though we cannot make our sun
Stand still, yet we will make him run!'
by Andrew Marvell, in *To His Coy Mistress*

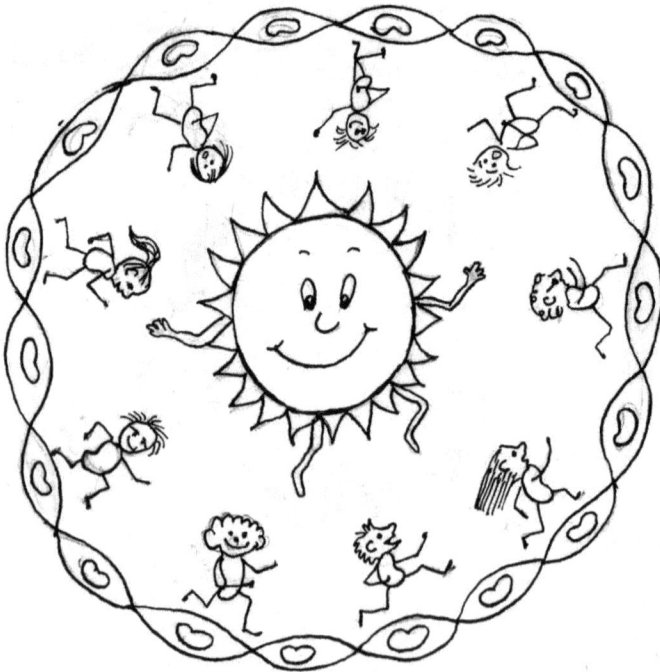

13

Should you learn to walk, before you can run?

Everything I wrote about exercise in the previous chapter applies to running. I may be biased – well, I am biased – but I believe running is the exercise Nature intended us to take. Our bodies are made for it, in spite of all our attempts to unmake them. If you can recapture even a little of the joy you experienced from running as a child, do it!

The only note of warning I would sound is that, if you are coming back to running after a number of years of not running, listen carefully to your body. Stretch your muscles a little and warm them up before you go out. Strengthen your legs gradually, paying close attention to any warning niggles or pains you may feel in your knees, hips and ankles. They may just be passing discomforts that your joints and muscles will go through, as they re-acclimatise to unaccustomed exertion, but they may also be messages that you should receive, acknowledge and act on.

Most people are sensible enough to stretch their muscles before exercise, but many forget to stretch them again afterwards. It's understandable: if you've worked your body hard, you naturally feel entitled to a rest. However, your muscles will probably stretch much more effectively, when they are warm. This is the stretching session that helps to reduce post-exercise stiffness.

Indeed, some runners advocate having your main stretching session after the first mile or so, once your muscles start to warm up.

If you demur at the phrase 'first mile or so', adjust it to the sort of distance you think you can run without too much trouble. As with all exercise programs, it's very important not to overdo the effort in the first flush of enthusiasm.

I once watched one of the greatest Olympic athletes working out in a gym. He was famous for his strength and stamina and had won gold medals at several Games, so I was curious to see how he trained. To my surprise, he hardly seemed to be trying at all, pressing and stretching with weights almost casually, exchanging a few friendly words with other athletes – but he kept going. There was none of the urgency I had seen in him when he was competing, but his body was moving freely, easily, well within its capacity. That, I am sure, is the quality that enabled him to keep competing at the highest level for more years than most observers thought possible. Remember: you're not trying to win medals. You're making a long-term investment in your body. Look after it.

Starting from scratch

If you are going to rely on running, walking and/or cycling as your main regular exercise, your aim will probably be to complete four or five sessions per week. For someone already reasonably fit, a run of 5-6km requires about the same effort as a brisk walk of about 10-12km or a bicycle ride of about 20-25km. To keep things interesting, it's a good idea to vary your routes and your schedule, doing at least one run, one walk and one cycle ride each week. If you don't already have a program of regular exercise, build up the days and the distance gradually.

If you haven't been out running since God was a boy, be very gentle with yourself. First of all, make sure you have the right shoes. Go out early in the morning, if you don't want to your neighbours to see what you're doing. Set yourself manageable targets. Try running from one streetlamp to the next. How did that feel? Allow yourself to walk to the next streetlamp, while you recover your breath, then jog gently to the next one, and so on. For the first outing, half a dozen streetlamps may be enough – or 8, 10 or 12. You may be fit enough to run for two or three streetlamps at a time. Or you may run the length of one street and then walk the next. It's your program. Its sole purpose is to help and benefit your body. No pressure. Take it easy.

Whatever the distance, when you feel you've done enough, go home. Have a rest, do some warming-down stretches, take a shower or a bath and congratulate yourself. You have just taken the first steps on what may be a long journey back to the health and energy levels you had as a child. Try to do something similar tomorrow, and the next day, and the next day. As ever, listen to your body, but keep going.

If your muscles are stiff, stretch them some more or have a massage; if you have blisters on your feet, give them the treatment they need. Change your shoes or socks, go cycling instead of walking or running and give them time to get better – but keep taking some sort of exercise – every day, if possible – or, failing that, every other day, but at least two or three times a week.

Just as you keep a daily record of your progress toward your target weight, you may like to measure and time your runs, with a Fitbit, an iPhone or similar. Don't be too competitive about it: this is not a race, but you will probably observe a marked improvement, as the weeks and months go by. It's another useful way of testing that the program you have set yourself is really beginning to make a difference.

Keep on running

Where running was concerned, our prehistoric forebears had it easy. Look at the motivation they had: they were either running to secure a delicious dinner for themselves and their families, or they were running to avoid becoming the delicious dinner of some other, fiercer creature. No wonder it was a case of survival of the fittest: only the fastest and strongest made the cut. Lacking those life and death imperatives, how can we offer ourselves the motivation we need, to push our soft, over-indulged bodies to new heights of athleticism?

Exhilaration is one way. Once you have got past the first month or so of your regular running program, when those initially stiff muscles have hardened up a little, and you're beginning to enjoy at least parts of your self-imposed regime, give yourself a break. I don't mean take a day or two off running – quite the contrary: head for the longest, open, downhill slope you can find, grassy or sandy if possible, get yourself to the top of it, and start to run down it, as fast as you can comfortably go.

Let yourself feel the slope and gravity carrying you along, faster than you could ever run on the flat, with surprisingly little effort on your part, other than trying to stay upright. Isn't that a glorious sensation? It's the sort of feeling you only experience if you run on an almost daily basis. It makes all your hard work seem suddenly worthwhile.

Other motivations include feeling fitter and healthier than you have felt for years and realising that your exercise plan really does help you to lose weight, when used in tandem with your reducing diet plan. Then, of course, there is the possibility of impressing your friends…

Some years ago, I rather rashly entered a Sydney Morning Herald Half-Marathon. After 17km, I was thinking about slowing from a stumble to a walk for a few moments, to gather my strength for the final assault – or so I told myself – when I spotted a hand-made sign, held by a spectator. It read '4km to go – and bragging rights forever!' First, it made me smile – no mean feat, in the circumstances – and then it persuaded me to keep on running, right to the finish line. And they were right about the bragging, as you may have noticed.

'The fault, dear Brutus, is not in our stars,
But in ourselves…'
Cassius, trying to persuade Brutus to join the conspiracy
against Caesar, in *Julius Caesar*, Act 1, Scene 2,
by William Shakespeare

'Our remedies oft in ourselves do lie,
Which we ascribe to heaven.'
Helena, deciding to take her destiny into her own hands,
in *All's Well that Ends Well*, Act 1, Scene 1,
by William Shakespeare

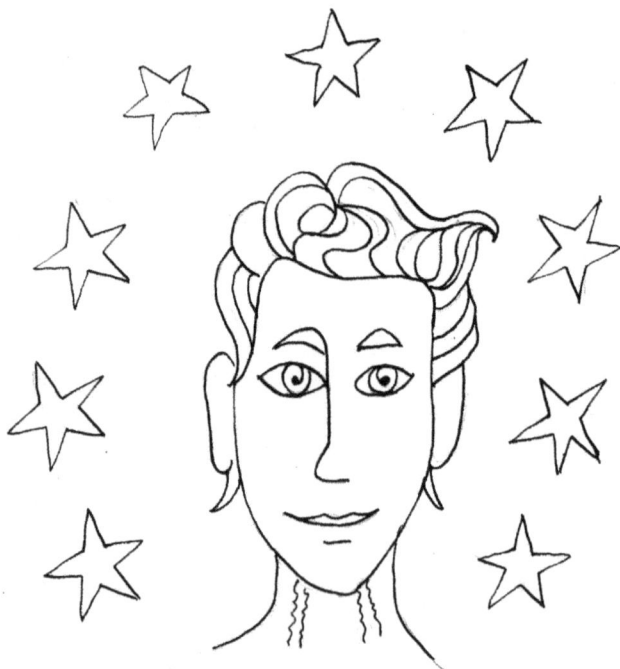

14

Why worry about cholesterol?

There is nothing wrong with cholesterol. All animals produce it and it performs vital functions in our bodies. Excessive cholesterol, however, is a serious and very common problem, which can lead to strokes, heart attacks and other health problems. Why not get your levels tested?

There are two types of cholesterol. Low Density Lipoprotein (LDL) is known as 'bad' cholesterol, because it leads to the build-up of plaque inside your blood vessels. This can harden and narrow your arteries and restrict the flow of blood – sometimes fatally. The other type, High Density Lipoprotein (HDL) is considered 'good' cholesterol, because it carries the LDL to your liver, which removes it from your blood system.

In the USA, the Centers for Disease Control and Prevention estimate that almost one-third of the entire population has unacceptably high levels of LDL. The probability increases with age: only 22% of people in their twenties have it; for those in their fifties, the figure rises to 62%.

There are other factors to consider, when calculating your chances. For example, anyone who is sufficiently interested in booze, cheese and chocolate to read – or write – a book about them probably has a fair chance of suffering this diet-related condition! That's enough bad news: the good news is that you can do something about it.

Your doctor is likely to advise you to take statins. They are said to have few side-effects (although some people suffer muscle pain and fatigue) – but once you have started taking them, you will probably have to continue for the rest of your life. If you're happy about that, feel free to skip the rest of this chapter. But, for someone with your strength of willpower and determination, there is an alternative.

If you have high levels of LDL cholesterol, as well as wishing to reduce your weight, it makes a lot of sense to tackle both problems at the same time. The recommended foods are not all identical, but there is a considerable overlap. If you are going to commit to a weight-reduction plan, why not cut back your cholesterol level at the same time?

It's not simply a matter of avoiding foods containing a lot of cholesterol. Saturated fats can also raise your cholesterol levels, so you need to limit foods containing them, as well as not smoking (of course!), reducing your alcohol intake to boost liver function and taking plenty of exercise.

Foods you should cut down or out

All animal products contain cholesterol; all plant foods do not. Animal foods also contain saturated fats, while plant foods contain little or none, with the exception of tropical oils such as coconut-based foods and the dreaded palm oil. Some foods, eggs, liver, kidneys and shellfish are high in cholesterol but low in saturated fats, so they may be included in your diet, to add variety and valuable nutrients, but in moderate amounts.

To reduce LDL cholesterol, cut down on saturated fats from animal products. If you love meat, look for less fatty cuts, preferably grass-fed, because the oil profile is better.

Foods you should reduce significantly

All dairy products – milk, cream, butter, high-fat cheeses
Tropical oils, coconut and particularly palm oil
All meats and meat products, especially if they are grain-fed and have a high fat content
Takeaways and all foods cooked in cheap, partially hydro-genated vegetable oils, which contain dangerous trans fats.
Pies, pastries, croissants, cakes, biscuits, snack bars, puddings
Chips, crisps, salted nuts, most processed foods
Sugar and white flour.

Foods you can enjoy with a clear conscience and clear arteries

All vegetables, raw in salads or lightly cooked
All fruit, raw or cooked, but be wary of sugary fruits, eg watermelon
Oily fish – preferably line-caught and sustainable, is a wonderful source of Omega 3
All fresh fish. Tinned fish after checking for additives
Pulses: beans, lentils, chick peas, soybeans, quinoa, tofu
Olive oil, pref. extra virgin – raises HDL but watch calories
Unsweetened almond milk or oat or soy milk instead of dairy milk
Low-fat yoghurts in place of ice cream
Sunflower, pumpkin & sesame seeds, sprinkled on salads.

Foods you can enjoy with some circumspection

Breads, cereals, rice, pasta (but watch the calories!)

All raw nuts (in moderation because of calories)

Cheeses: cottage, quark, part-skim ricotta or mozzarella, low-fat cheddar and others. Save high-fat cheeses for special occasions. Portion control is essential. Read the labels carefully!

Small quantities of very lean, grass-fed meats

Chicken breast without skin

Chocolate, preferably dark and made with as little milk and sugar as possible – bearing in mind the previous advice on quantities.

Moral Fibre

Foods containing soluble fibre reduce cholesterol and LDL levels. Oatmeal and oat bran are outstanding, whether raw or cooked. Kidney beans, apples, pears, prunes and even sweet potato and potato skins all contain useful amounts of soluble fibre.

Fishy Fats

Unlike fatty meats, fatty fish can be highly beneficial to heart health, because they contain significant amounts of omega-3 fatty acids, which can improve your blood flow, thin the blood (reducing the risk of blood clots forming) and help to regulate the electrical signalling of the heart. Oily fish like sardines, anchovies, herring, mackerel, trout, salmon and tuna are preferred to white fish, because they feed further from the seafloor – but large, deep-sea predators also have an unfortunate tendency to carry higher levels of contaminants like mercury and dioxins.

Eating these species of fish two or three times a week will give you a useful amount of omega-3 fatty acids. Omega-3s don't lower cholesterol but they do reduce triglycerides, another marker of heart health. Some dietitians recommend taking an additional teaspoon or so of premium quality fish oil for this reason. Quality is important and can be measured by the amounts of omega-3 acids, eicosapentaenoic acid (EPA) and docosohexaenoic acid (DHA) in the oil. Check with your physician first in case of any impact on other medication.

Nutty fats

Nuts are another valuable source of polyunsaturated fatty acids. They should be raw, rather than roasted, and free from added sugar or salt. As nuts are heavy on calories, just have a small quantity every day. Imagine a golf ball made of nuts – and pour them into a small bowl, rather than helping yourself more liberally from the jar or packet!

A holistic approach

Everything you do to lose weight will also tend to reduce your cholesterol levels – exercise will improve your overall fitness and blood flow and reduce your body fat. Reducing stress, caffeine and alcohol can all be helpful at times. It's a delicate balancing act, where the aim is to achieve a personal regime that will be beneficial without punishing yourself. If you can get into the habit of listening to your body, your True Self will probably tell you what's best for you. Just don't let Greedy Self interrupt!

'Doc, note, I dissent: a fast never prevents a fatness.
I diet on cod'
   – a stunning palindrome (word or phrase whose letters
read the same backwards as forwards). It was invented
by Peter Hilton, one of the famous code-breakers who
cracked the German Enigma code at Bletchley Park in
World War Two.

It's brilliant but inaccurate, because a well-timed fast
can indeed prevent a fatness. This version is six letters
shorter but I prefer it because it also conveys a valuable
piece of advice:
'Doc, note, I dissent: a fast reverts a fatness. I diet on cod'

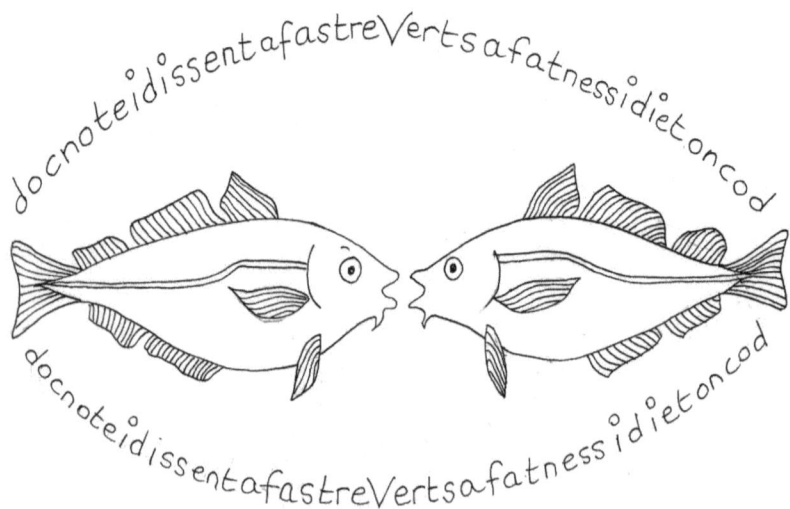

15

What else do you need?

What you need, above all, to succeed with any diet plan is the willpower and determination I mentioned in the last chapter. Unless you're a bit stubborn and bloody-minded, you won't succeed, so it's worth doing whatever you can to cultivate those qualities – but try not to let them spill over into the rest of your family life!

One thing you can easily do, to strengthen your resolve, is keep accurate records of your progress – on bad days as well as good ones. When you look back over a few weeks or months, you'll be able to see exactly when you made progress and when you slipped back a little.

If you have the time, it's a good idea to keep an accurate log of what you eat, each day, and count the calories. In my experience, few people are organised enough to keep that going over a long period. So try to keep, at least, minimal records of your progress every day.

Let's say you decide to have five different diet plans:

F FASTING – up to 800 calories per day

R REDUCING – less than 1,500 calories per day

M MAINTAINING – around 2,000 calories per day

I INDULGING – up to 3,000 calories per day

P PIGGING OUT – (rarely) you may hit 4,000-5,000 calories in a day

First thing in the morning, weigh yourself and write it down. Then, write what diet plan you are intending to follow for that day: **F**, **R**, **M**, **I** or **P**. Then, write what amount of exercise you intend to take, running, cycling, weights, tennis, etc., and how long you plan to spend on it. Finally, fill in the diet plan and exercise routine you actually followed for the previous day. You will find this goes a long way towards explaining the apparently mysterious ups and downs of your weight.

There are other factors, such as temporary fluid retention, that may explain small variations in weight, but over time, this simple record will tell its own story. Armed with this accurate information, you will be able to make informed decisions. If you have one or two social events coming up, where you know you will be indulging or feasting, why not pave the way with a day or two of fasting or reducing? That way, you will set yourself free to enjoy those days with a clear conscience. If you miss the chance to cut back before the parties, you can always do so later – but it never feels quite so good, paying back the calories after the feast.

A Personal Note

Since you've read this far, let me explain that I'm not asking anyone to try and do something I haven't done myself. I don't underestimate the degree of difficulty in sticking to a weight reducing and/or cholesterol lowering diet – but I know that the personal rewards for success are greater than for almost anything else you could do.

I've had slightly high cholesterol since I was in my thirties – quite a long time ago, now. About ten years ago,

I'd been in a sedentary job for a few years. I hadn't been taking enough exercise, and my weight had gone up to almost 100kg. My doctor suggested – and I agreed – that it was about time I did something about both problems. I said I'd prefer not to start taking statins, if I could avoid it. He suggested I should enlist the help of a dietitian, Dr Naras Lapsys, who has generously helped me to write this book – indeed, it would never have existed, but for his wise counsel.

Rather than setting a fixed regime for me to follow, Naras first questioned me closely about what I wanted to achieve, in terms of weight loss and cholesterol reduction. Then he asked about what and when I like to eat and drink. Together, we fashioned a diet plan that I thought I could achieve. I went back to see him again, three or four times over the next few months, and we checked my progress and modified the plan accordingly. After six months or so, my weight was not far over 80kg, my cholesterol was not low, but acceptable, and I surprised myself by running my first Sydney Half-Marathon in a reasonable time.

I had tried to lose weight before, but with disappointing results. I found I got bored with the regime before achieving my targets – and I resented 'being told what to do' – even though I was actually telling myself to do it. I realised that, for a diet to work, the person dieting must own the plan and feel in control of what's happening. That's why I haven't been too specific about exactly what you should eat and when: my guess is that you wouldn't be able to stick to an imposed regime for very long, because, like me, you need to feel that it's your own choice.

Many people say breakfast is 'the most important meal of the day' but I prefer to skip breakfast in favour of lunch, where I will often have a bowl of rolled oats and steel-cut oats with a sprinkling of oat bran, with cinnamon for flavour. I pour hot (not boiling) water on this, just short of covering it, and add a topping of fruit or a tablespoon or two of really good muesli or granola (not too much and not too sugary) and then pour on some fresh, unsweetened almond milk. These are low glycemic index foods (apart from the topping) which sustain you for longer because they release energy slowly. Any other low glycemic foods would do as well.

Solving the cholesterol problem

I'd been aware of my high cholesterol levels for years. I knew that it could lead to the formation of plaques that would build up inside my arteries, over time, and that this could reduce my blood flow with ultimately serious or even catastrophic consequences – but, being a natural optimist, I told myself it could never happen to me.

I now understand that the process is much more complicated than that. Cholesterol doesn't actually form plaques. LDL particles carry cholesterol and fats and get trapped in the linings of the blood vessels. They get oxidised and become inflamed. It's the inflammation that causes damage and over time soft plaques form. Then they harden and scarring develops. It's as if you had a terrible case of acne, inside your arteries. If only we could see it, we'd be much more determined to do something about it. And that, for me, was the breakthrough I needed.

Some years after my first successful weight loss, it became all too obvious that my weight had crept up again, not to 100kg, but around 90kg, which was about 8-10kg too much. My doctor suggested repeating the weight loss diet and also recommended a more detailed cholesterol test with a cardiologist, just to see how serious the problem was.

In the test, an electronic sensor next to my neck created a real-time image of the blood flowing through my carotid artery. I was surprised to see that the stream seemed to be about one-third filled with rocky debris. I asked the technician what it was. She told me it was plaque 'furring up' my arteries. Seeing this for myself made all the difference. Plaque build-up was no longer an abstract idea, to be dealt with at some time in the future, but real and immediate, in my own body, and visible. I'd seen my own internal acne – and realised that it could kill me.

In the ensuing consultation with the cardiologist, he explained that the arteries in my heart would almost certainly be in a similar condition. He recommended that I should start taking statins and transition to the highest dose, which, he thought, would just about get my cholesterol down to a safe level, and might even make some minor improvements.

I listened and nodded but was still stunned by what I had seen. I thought I'd have to be pretty stupid to ignore such a warning, but I was still reluctant to take statins. I know they are among the safest medications in the world, with remarkably few or minor side-effects, but I just wondered if there was another solution.

I decided to cut out all foods containing cholesterol for the next five months. Once again, my weight dropped to 80-82kg, I ran another Sydney Half-Marathon and, best of all, I had a blood test which showed my cholesterol was back in safe levels, with low LDL and high HDL.

I didn't want to spend the rest of my life avoiding meat, eggs, cheese and other dairy products altogether, so I decided to reintroduce them to my diet in moderation. To compensate for this self-indulgence, I check my weight every morning. When it goes over a certain level, I quickly go back on a reducing diet for a few days, to lose 2-3 kilos. I also get my blood tested regularly, to monitor my cholesterol levels. So far, so good.

I wouldn't completely rule out the idea of taking statins at some time in the future – I don't mean to demonise that medication, because it's a relatively risk-free way to preserve or lengthen life – but if so, it will be my choice and an informed one. Maybe I'm more stubborn than most people – my nearest and dearest certainly think so – but I like to feel in charge of my own body. And I still enjoy booze, cheese and chocolate!

Almond Milk

Various nut, soy and oat milks are readily available on supermarket shelves, if you want an alternative to dairy milk. They are all free from cholesterol but, of course, they contain various additives to preserve them for several months, and many brands contain a surprisingly low percentage of almonds. Personally, I prefer to make my own almond milk. It keeps in the refrigerator for about five days.

Here's how:

Soak 250g of (preferably organic) almonds in water overnight. This washes off the enzymes that delay sprouting, so after eight hours or so, your nuts are softer – a sprouting superfood. Rinse them clean, put them in a blender, add water to make one litre, and blend for about 90 seconds. Strain the mixture through a nut milk bag (available from good health stores) and add a quarter of a teaspoonful of vanilla or almond essence to taste, if you wish. The litre of milk will be delicious and don't throw away the almond meal, because someone who is not on a weight loss diet may like to make a cake or an apple crumble with it!

If you like, rinse the sprouted almonds in hot water and it will be fairly easy to rub off the skins. The milk will be a little clearer and will last a day or two longer in the refrigerator.

A final thought – tantric wine and cheese

If you find tantric chocolate works for you – and I hope you will – why not try the same trick with wine and cheese?

Try pouring your wine into a shot glass or liqueur glass. Don't knock it back in one: drink it in two or three mouthfuls. It will taste just as good as a big swig, especially if you savour it and don't swallow it too soon. Refill the shot glass as often as you like: you'll probably find you drink much less, in the course of a meal.

And if that works, try serving yourself much smaller portions of cheese. They will also taste just as good, if you don't wash them down too quickly. Portion control will reduce your total intake and allow you to eat cheese more often, albeit in smaller quantities.

Further Reading

It's really not possible to write anything in the weight loss dieting area without acknowledging Dr Michael Mosley, the science presenter, journalist, tv producer and now best-selling author of numerous books. Dr Mosley has done so much groundbreaking work in this area in recent years, that he has effectively made the field his own.

Then, why add to the flood of diet advice books? Simply because there are so many millions of us who could be happier and healthier and live longer, more fulfilling lives – if only we could eat and drink more wisely. There are as many diet plans as there are people in the world: it's a matter of finding the one that suits YOU and then sticking to it – or coming back to it, if and when you lapse into self-indulgence.

You don't have to give up every pleasure: if you like Booze, Cheese and Chocolate, you can include them in your new, healthy life-style – but you'll need to take control of what you eat and drink, do it mindfully and keep your goal in mind. Anything is possible. You can do this.

Much of the advice in this book has been influenced by Michael Mosley's pioneering work, from the original 5:2 diet, through the successful treatment and cure of diabetes (type 2) by dietary measures, to the Fast 800, where reducing the daily intake to 800 calories induces 'fat-burning' (ketosis) and significant weight loss in a surprisingly short period of time.

Mosley's many tv series are highly articulate, down-to-earth and easy to follow; his books are very similar. It's not rocket science, but it is very clever and it can help to transform people's lives.

The Fast Diet: the simple secret of intermittent fasting
by Michael Mosley and Mimi Spencer
The 5:2 Diet Book
by Kate Harrison, Orion (2013)
The 8 Week Blood Sugar Diet: how to beat diabetes fast and stay off medication
by Michael Mosley, Short Books Ltd. (revised edition, 2017)
The Clever Guts Diet: how to revolutionise your body from the inside out
by Michael Mosley, Short Books Ltd (2017)
The Fast 800: how to combine rapid weight loss and intermittent fasting for long-term health
by Michael Mosley, Short Books Ltd (2019)
Glucose Revolution: how to control your blood sugar levels to reduce inflammation-caused complaints and encourage natural weight loss, principally by eating foods in the right order
by Jessie Inchauspé, Simon & Schuster (2022)

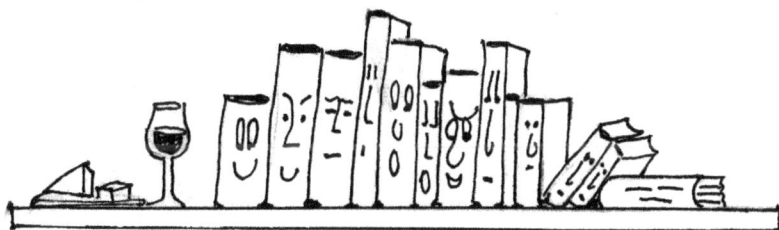

Calorie Counting

Losing weight is a numbers game and if you cheat, the only person you'll be cheating is yourself.

If you use less calories than you consume, your body will retain them and store them for later use, mainly as fat. If you use more calories than you consume, your body will supply the deficit from your stored fat.

If you find you're not losing weight as fast as you hoped, it will almost certainly be because you are overestimating the number of calories you use or underestimating the number of calories you consume. Simple.

If you are serious about losing weight, you need to know the calorific value of everything you eat and drink. Fortunately, this information is easy to find online.

There are many calorie counting websites from which to choose. An excellent one is calorieking.com.au which provides separate sites for Australia, UK and USA and measures the calories in most well-known brands and processed foods as well as fresh ingredients.

Apps to check calories online include easydietdiary and myfitnesspal but there are many others and most of them are free.

Valediction

'And whether we shall meet again, I know not.
Therefore our everlasting farewell take,
For ever, and for ever, fare well.
If we do meet again, why, we shall smile;
If not, why then, this parting was well made.'
Brutus to Cassius, as one conspirator to another,
in *Julius Caesar*, Act 5, Scene 1, by William Shakespeare.

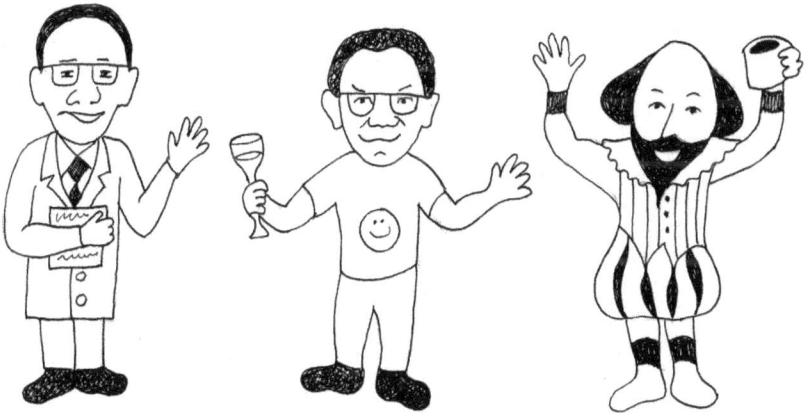

Progress Charts

	Start Date	Start Weight	Finish Date	Target Weight
Phase 1	_____	_____	_____	_____
Phase 2	_____	_____	_____	_____
Phase 3	_____	_____	_____	_____
Phase 4	_____	_____	_____	_____
Phase 5	_____	_____	_____	_____

Diet Plan Codes

F FASTING – up to 800 calories per day

R REDUCING – less than 1,500 calories per day

M MAINTAINING – around 2,000 calories per day

I INDULGING – up to 3,000 calories per day

P PIGGING OUT – (rarely) you may hit 4,000 - 5,000 calories in a day

Exercise Plan Codes

1 REST

2 LIGHT WORKOUT eg brisk walk

3 MODERATE EXERCISE

4 ENERGETIC

5 TO THE MAX

Daily Progress Charts

Phase _____   Week _____

Date	Morning Weight	Diet Plan	Actual Diet	Exercise Plan	Actual Exercise

Date	Morning Weight	Diet Plan	Actual Diet	Exercise Plan	Actual Exercise

Daily Progress Charts

Phase _____   Week _____

Date	Morning Weight	Diet Plan	Actual Diet	Exercise Plan	Actual Exercise

Date	Morning Weight	Diet Plan	Actual Diet	Exercise Plan	Actual Exercise

Daily Progress Charts

Phase _____   Week _____

Date	Morning Weight	Diet Plan	Actual Diet	Exercise Plan	Actual Exercise

Date	Morning Weight	Diet Plan	Actual Diet	Exercise Plan	Actual Exercise

Daily Progress Charts

Phase _____   Week _____

Date	Morning Weight	Diet Plan	Actual Diet	Exercise Plan	Actual Exercise

Date	Morning Weight	Diet Plan	Actual Diet	Exercise Plan	Actual Exercise